Age Gracefully: Make the Right Decisions for Your Skin

Dr. Chau Phan
Pharmacist and owner
of Pleasant Care Pharmacy

DEDICATION

I would like to dedicate this book to my two beautiful sons, Hieu and Khang. Hieu has had eczema since he was born, and with his condition now under control, he is well on his way to having healthy skin, just as his brother does.

CONTENTS

FOREWORD

Aging is an inevitable process that we must all eventually accept. Sometimes we may feel as though we're fighting a never-ending battle against our skin, and sometimes we may just want to wave the white flag and admit defeat. But we don't have to.

In this book, Dr. Chau Phan explains the causes of aging skin, which are important in understanding how to prevent and treat the signs. The proliferation of products and advertisements for anti-aging skin care is overwhelming, and a consumer who tries every miracle product that comes along will find the process pricey. Dr. Phan explains the changes we can make in our lives that will not only positively affect our skin, but our health in general. She also describes the ingredients that we should be using and why, so we can make the right decisions in choosing products that will save us money and give us the results we want.

Dr. Phan and I are alumnae of Thomas J. Long School of Pharmacy and Health Sciences. After I learned about the skin care products she creates, I sought her expertise for my father's skin ailment. For years he had been using a steroid prescription product for itchy skin. The relief was short term, and he kept refilling his medication. Because there are adverse effects to long-term use of steroids, I didn't want my father to continue using a product containing steroids as an active ingredient, especially when it wasn't improving his condition. Dr. Phan supplied him with one of her products, and he hasn't complained about his itchy skin since.

Dr. Phan's passion for assisting in the improvement of our skin is evident in this book. Even though we can't stop the aging process, her comprehensive explanation of how to care for our skin shows us a way to ease the struggle. With this information, we can throw down the white flag, face the inevitable with confidence, and age gracefully.

– Annie Patel, Pharm.D., Ph.D.

INTRODUCTION

The purpose of this book is to:

1. Bring to light the struggle to find the right skincare regimen

2. Teach people the basics of healthy skin and the causes of aging skin

3. Show others how to prevent skin from aging before it starts

4. Share ways to reverse the signs of aging skin

5. Educate people on how to choose products that meet their unique needs and provide a simple stepwise skincare approach that people can use themselves and teach others

CHAPTER 1: BRINGING TO LIGHT THE STRUGGLE TO FIND THE RIGHT SKINCARE REGIMEN

My own struggle

I was born and raised in Saigon, Vietnam and lived there until the age of ten years old. It was right after the Vietnam War, so everyone was grappling with the change in regime and trying to find stability and food to eat. Skincare or skin protection was the last thing on anyone's mind. Even though Vietnam is a hot and humid country, no one was using anything for their skin.

Sunscreen was non-existent in Vietnam and only really a consideration when I first moved to America for use when I was going to spend a full day in the sun, such as going to the beach or swimming in a pool. My family was very poor, so we did not have set skincare regimens. Therefore, I was not using anything until I started college.

By then, I heard from a friend that you needed to wear sunscreen every day, but, for everyday use, I could only afford to buy moisturizer with SPF 15. That was my daily regimen until I was thirty years old. By then, I had already become a pharmacist and started noticing fine lines around my eyes. I wanted to do something about that, so I started looking into skincare.

It was around this time that I saw an infomercial about a skincare product endorsed by a supermodel. The infomercial showed that the product helped the supermodel maintain her beautiful skin because the product contains a rare melon extract only found in a remote region in the south of France. The results were there for everyone to see on the screen. I had just started to see the signs of aging on my skin and thought I needed a magic solution like that to counteract it. I thought that this might be the breakthrough for me. I thought to myself, "If someone this beautiful could get results like this from a bottle, maybe it will work for me." Also, this rare melon extract only found in France sounded so mysterious that I wanted to try it.

So I picked up the phone, ready to order. The representative on the phone then told me that the product would be sent to me automatically every month, and she wanted my credit card number. I stopped dead in my tracks and asked myself, "What are you doing?!? You are a pharmacist and researcher. You need to do research to find out what the best ingredient is for your own skin. Don't listen to this infomercial!" I kindly declined to give the representative my credit card number and hung up the phone.

After that, I started my own journey of research: reading reports on various clinical trials, reviewing articles, learning the basics of skin. When I got a sense of what causes skin to age and which ingredients can help avoid or reverse the aging process, it became apparent that I needed to find products that contain anti-aging ingredients.

This was a huge challenge because there are so many products to choose from, and most skincare providers do not tell you how much of any ingredient they put into their products. This made it difficult for me to pick the right product for my skin. I could see the different ingredients that I wanted for my skin but struggled to find them all in one place. This meant that I would have to buy more than one product to get all the ingredients that I wanted.

Because I am a low-maintenance person who wants to keep the number of creams I put on my skin to a minimum (ideally, one!), I opted for the best ingredient for my skin and chose only one product to use.

I encountered another challenge when I saw that the ingredient I wanted was in several different brands. The cost of the products varied greatly even though they all contained the same ingredients. After looking through the different brands, I opted for the one with the most favorable reviews and that seemed the most legitimate.

The horrors of choosing the wrong skincare

Choosing the right skincare is one thing, but what can be even scarier is choosing the wrong products for your skin. Personally, I don't have any horror stories about choosing the wrong product. Maybe that's because I don't have sensitive skin, and I also don't like to try a lot of products. However, after years of helping people with their skin problems, I have encountered many horror stories about people choosing the wrong products.

Recently, I met someone at the tender age of 21 who had been experimenting with different skincare products and cosmetics, trying to find the right ones for her. She was taking advantage of the free samples offered from many places – in the mail, online, in stores and with magazines. She put one of these free samples on her skin and it caused her skin to break out. And, even though she stopped applying that particular sample, she did not recover from the acne it caused.

Not knowing how to resolve her acne, she started popping her pimples, thinking that she could get rid of the acne that way. Now, the acne had spread from her cheeks to the rest of her face and then to her body. As you can see from her story, having sensitive skin can pose a danger when you are trying out different products – especially when you have not done the research and you do not know what is in them.

Another case involved a patient of mine, who, at the age of 60, decided that she should look for a new skincare product to help her as she got older. The product made her face peel, caused redness and irritation, and left her skin sensitive to sunlight. Due to the sensitivity to sunlight, she started getting dark spots on her face. This, in turn, motivated her to purchase yet another cream to get rid of the dark spots, but the cream made her face even darker. Her face was now very thin and so sensitive, she could not tolerate alcohol on it. The stinging made her scared to try anything new on her face.

That initial decision of hers – to change her skin regimen – caused her to have sensitive skin for the rest of her life. The point here is that, once someone has had a bad experience, it can potentially ruin his or her skin for life and cause a lack of openness to trying anything new.

However, this closed attitude will keep someone like her from having the opportunity to find what's right for her skin.

I want to help people be confident in how they look so that they feel better about themselves and the "face" they present to the rest of the world. That is why I promote self-education and partner with my clients to discover the ingredients that work best for them. The benefit of this approach is that you are working with someone credentialed in pharmacology who can help you avoid losing money, and worse, damaging your skin during the discovery process.

Another patient I had was a 40-year-old woman who had dry skin and a little bit of acne on her chin. Because she is someone who networks frequently, she met many women who sell skincare products from multi-level marketing skincare companies. These women started to push her to use their products and claimed that their products would help her. She trusted them and tried their products.

Not only did this approach not help her, it made her face drier than it had been before, and her acne got worse. She relied on these women because she trusted them, but they were a part of a multi-level marketing scheme. They are there to sell products and make a commission, not help her. My point is this: I could tell many more horror stories than I have room for in this book, but all the stories have a common thread: **Not knowing what to use and experimenting without information specific to your needs is dangerous to your skin's health. I can help.**

The influence of media and marketing on what we pay for skincare

Recently, I did a little research to see the different choices and price ranges for skincare. I entered a high-end department store and spent some time checking out the different skincare lines there. I went in with an open mind and was greeted by an assistant who asked what I was looking for. After a brief consultation, the first cream she recommended was in the price range of around $370. Even given the high-end nature of the store I was shopping in, I found the price surprising.

I explained that this was over my budget and that I was looking for something at a lower price point. The assistant asked me what my price range was. This set me back a little because the assistant should be recommending something that is good for me and my specific skincare needs, rather than any product that fits into my price range. She then quickly recommended a cream under $100 as an alternative. When I compared the ingredients listed on the two products, I found not much difference between the two. The less expensive cream the salesperson recommended was less than a third of the price of the first recommendation and had ingredients that would have a similar effect on my skin.

At the studio where I record my Vietnamese talk show, "Pharmacy in Our Lives", while waiting for my turn to record, I met a woman who asked to buy some cream. First, I asked her, "Are you looking to buy ice cream? I don't think they sell ice cream at the studio." She chuckled and said, "No, I want to buy anti-aging face cream."

It turns out that the recording studio also sells anti-aging cream from Asia. This was a larger size than the $370 product I had seen at the high-end department store and only cost somewhere in the region of $30. I found that the ingredients in this cream were very similar to the ones in that $370 product. I saw this as an example of how we can be easily misled into making wrong choices. The high-end store with the immaculate cosmetics counter and the well-groomed and well-trained staff member is very reassuring. They make you believe that you are buying into a solution and a specific lifestyle.

But when you look past all of the marketing, you can tell that you are not buying all the hoopla. At the base level, the product you're purchasing is a mixture of ingredients that, when put together in a jar, can have a particular effect on your skin. Those ingredients are what you should be looking at. Those ingredients as listed on the side of the jar are often the same no matter whether they were put together by a big company or a local producer.

Finding the right skincare can be a real struggle! We have all tried and tested many skin creams during our life, only to find that the magic formula that will solve all our skincare problems eludes us. As if there were a magic potion that **could** solve everyone's individual skincare issues!

The marketers perpetuate the myth that such a magic potion exists, and they have even, maybe, been successful in getting us to think that the issues their product solves are ones we have identified and experienced ourselves (even though, often, those issues are not our issues). Sometimes, we are naïve enough to believe the myth, so we buy their cream and become victims of their false advertising.

Marketing has changed the way we lead our lives, behave as consumers and view ourselves. We are cajoled into thinking that certain solutions will change the way we are, the way we feel and the way we are viewed by others. In this society, we no longer buy just products. We buy solutions. We buy a better life. We buy a new lifestyle. We buy acceptance. And when we "buy" all of these intangibles, we convince ourselves (with a little help from the advertisers) that we also buy the envy of our neighbors, friends and family.

The marketing departments of big companies have years of experience in how to separate us from our hard-earned money. They know our weak spots! The advent of the internet and social media has also changed the game, and not necessarily in the consumer's favor. It has made it even easier to spread more information and speak to more people on a smaller budget.

Skincare is like any other business – it is designed to make money from consumers. Yet, I am not advocating a boycott of skincare products or anything like that. There will always be products that will help you in your quest to look better and feel better about yourself.

Remember: Anti-aging is not a pipe dream. It can happen. But what you need to know is that the company with the biggest marketing budget or the highest sales is not necessarily the right one for you. Nor is the company with the smallest budget either, for that matter. Many other factors are at play here than just how much it costs to produce and market a product. Most importantly, in the case of skincare, your health should be your chief consideration. So don't be sucked in by big-budget ads or celebrity endorsements. Look further into the products, based on your needs.

Think about the last beauty or fashion magazine you read. If it's anything like the last one I read, it will consist of around 40 percent advertisements. In there will also be features about the latest skincare regimen, the greatest diet to ever be discovered and interviews with the most beautiful movie and TV stars.

It's all about extending the sale of a lifestyle. Somewhere deep down in your psyche you are reading these magazines because you want to be like these people. You want to have some part of the lifestyle depicted on their pages. You may not want to be a movie star, but you may want the level of glamor, attention, and income being portrayed on the pages of the magazine.

Sitting alongside these tempting views of what life could be like among the rich and famous are feature articles about how to grow old gracefully, how to eat the right foods for your skin, how to lose 20 pounds in a month, and what to wear when you have achieved all of these other things. It's a total package they have put together: The articles tell us "Be like these people in the stories, and follow all of our advice, and you, too, will become glamorous, rich and famous."

And that's before the 40 percent of advertisements kicks in. They add to the illusion that all you have to do is follow **their** advice and buy **their** products, and you will get to this place you want to be. You reason to yourself that, if the magazine is there to help you get to the hallowed land of a skinnier, healthier, more beautiful you, the advertisements must be for products that can do that too, right?

Remember: Nothing beats doing your own research and saying "no" to what is not best for you.

The first rule of making smart skincare choices is clear. Acknowledge that there are many reasons we want to look great: feeling great, having greater access to a promotion at work, a better chance of finding a partner, maybe even being approached in the street and offered a modeling job. Understand that the benefits of looking better and younger are based on vanity, something we are all subject to. The advertising and product packaging play to this weakness in all of us.

Remember: Your skin in reality does not have the benefit of airbrushing. In real life, you can never achieve the perfection of the superstar's airbrushed looks, and you will always be left in disappointment when it comes to attempting to recreate that look for yourself.

Another tactic advertisers use is before and after photos. In the before photo, their subject's skin is made to look as though it's in worse shape than it was at the time the picture was taken. They then take an after photo with great lighting, maybe a digital touch-up or two and then publish the ad. In this way, they have pricked your vanity, and you will often fall for it. You think, "If that can help her, then it will help me too."

Remember: Your vanity is not the right part of your being to help you make these purchase decisions about which anti-aging skin cream will work for you.

A more modern technique in advertising is to roll out an A-List celebrity to tell consumers what a great product it is that they're pitching. Just a quick Google search will bring up scores of celebrity endorsements for skincare products.

This technique ties in with what we have discussed earlier with respect to magazine and TV advertising. Even if the celebrities in these advertisements don't actually say that they use the product themselves, they certainly hint that the products they're pitching worked for them. Again, our subconscious tells us that, if it got them their acting career, billionaire husband or that house in Malibu, then it can work for us.

Remember: You are not buying the chance to be the next Beyonce. You are not buying a shot at being in a movie. You are buying a selection of ingredients that, together, may or may not have the effect on your skin that you are looking for.

Product positioning and packaging and how they influence us

Many products, especially in cosmetics and skincare, appear in carefully chosen places in the stores where they are sold. When you walk into your local store and Brand A is within your line of sight and framed by an attractive, set-apart display area, you are immediately drawn to it; that is no coincidence. That space has been sold to the manufacturer by the retailer.

Meanwhile, Brand B sits on the bottom shelf, often overlooked because the company that produces it couldn't come up with the cash to secure a more prominent spot.

Linked to the product's placement in the store is the quality of the packaging and how it looks on the shelf. These factors get your mind to imagine how it would look in your bathroom. The big companies with the big budgets can afford to spend a little more on a box to go around their jar of cream. The box will be made of quality cardboard and printed in vibrant colors.

All of this together makes you believe that you are buying the best quality you can. Great packaging and a high price point are great indicators of quality if you don't know how to look at the ingredients and make a decision based on what the cream can actually do for you.

Remember: The cream on the bottom shelf in the less fancy packaging may have more efficacious ingredients better suited to your needs than Product A, on which the producer may has spent more money on packaging, advertising, and product placement than on what the product contains. Be your own best advocate and disregard the glitz and glamor. Your answer lies in what's inside.

Product properties versus ingredients' effects

Once we have been exposed to all the advertisements for a cream and listened to all the things that it can do for us, we start to think about the cream for what it actually is. But, again, we may not be educated enough to understand how the ingredients work, so we look at the properties of the cream instead.

One method people may use to choose a skin cream is by the way it feels on their skin. We attribute certain properties to the cream based on the way it feels when it is being applied. We call it rich, we call it soothing, we call it replenishing, and we call it light or any of a hundred other words.
Manufacturers and their marketers get to the core of how we want the cream to make us feel. They really reach out to what we want, or what we think we want, from a skincare product.

These descriptions of the product's properties mean very little when looked at in comparison with the effects of the ingredients, especially in terms of how those ingredients work together. So, we may experience the cream as rich, soothing, replenishing or light without any scientific or empirical evidence to back up that feeling.

Remember: You can actually find out what an ingredient does and how that relates to the way it makes your skin look and feel. This will really liberate your buying choices and help you hone in on what you should be looking for in a skincare product.

How changes in our skin affect skincare choices

Even when we find a product that we think works, its beneficial effects don't last forever. Your skin changes based on the season, the weather, your lifestyle and your age. When I speak to women, they often tell me that they think the product they started using years ago should continue to work the same way.

After all, they reason that it took them many tries to find that one product that worked for them. Shouldn't its positive effects continue even to today? Instead, they find that, after a short while, the product stops having the desired effect. They wonder why that is. Is it the formula? Is it something I've done or not done? Is it my diet?

Many factors influence how our skin looks, and the key to all of this is to understand what is going on. When you know what your skin is doing and what your skin needs, you will also know what to give it. You will know the ingredients to buy and the creams that contain them. But I suspect many of you are like I was – stuck in a struggle to find the right skincare and confused by the process.

Much of what underlies your purchase of a skincare product is the lifestyle element.

Remember: The lifestyle element **is** crucial in the selection of skincare and cosmetics – not the lifestyle of the rich and famous depicted in advertising, but the style of the life **we** are living. We have already seen how companies are prepared to pay huge sums of money to try to convince us that purchasing their products will get us linked in to the kind of life that celebrity has.

Beyonce's contract with L'Oreal for its hair care products was around $4 million for 10 days of work. That is an indication of how important what you are buying into is for the cosmetic companies. Think critically about your decisions: The choices you are making need to integrate with your life as **you** live it – with the food and beverages you ingest, the amount of exposure to the elements you experience, the number of hours of sleep you get on a regular basis, the supplements and medication you are taking.

Free samples – good, bad or indifferent?

Another way people make their skincare choices is to try the free samples from magazines and stores. These samples are often placed with advertisements so that you can "try before you buy". Trying the product there and then puts you in the position of going into the situation blind because you are putting something on your face that you have no information about. You may have allergies or sensitivities to certain ingredients. You don't want to have any negative effects be an after-the-fact ugly surprise!

Remember: You are responsible for what you apply to your skin. Avoid trying free samples until you have the opportunity to research and know what kind of ingredients are in the product first.

What's inside is what matters

Good quality ingredients should be at the core of the skincare product that will help you. As we have seen, quality ingredients can be found in the jar of cream that costs a few dollars as readily as they can be found in one that costs a few hundred dollars. The key is to know what to look for. Once you have this knowledge in your armory, you can make the decisions that are right for you.

But finding a product that has good quality ingredients is only half the battle. The other half is to know whether those good quality ingredients are actually good for your skin. That is where the education and advice contained in this book will really help you.

I can teach you how to read product labels and extract the information you need to make the right decisions for you. I can help you transform the way you look at skincare products and their packaging forever because you will know where to look and what to look for. You will look beyond the price, beyond the celebrity endorsements and beyond the fancy packaging.

You will understand how to go straight to the ingredients list to learn what you need to know.

What we've learned so far about the influence of marketing on our skincare choices

As you can see, there are many methods we use to select our skincare products in the quest to find something that slows the signs of aging. We can see that these methods are not based on science. Of course, the companies that sell these creams will tell you that they have been scientifically tested to produce certain results and that their customers love the creams.

In some cases, you will also be told that a certain celebrity really loves the cream as well. But relying on someone to do the research who is paid to sell a cream to you isn't doing right by you. They have a vested interest in selling the cream to you, so they are unlikely to provide you with a balanced view.

I am here to help you carry out your own research and find a product that is right for you and your skin. But don't worry; you won't need a science lab and a lot of expensive equipment to carry out this research. This book will teach you to look for the right ingredients that can help you and to find them in as inexpensive a form as possible.

You can slash the cost of your skincare regimen by understanding what to look for. You will be able to buy with confidence, knowing what the products will do rather than relying on the advertising to make the decisions for you. Once you are armed with information and education, you can make the choices that will help you on the road to growing old gracefully.

Skincare industry regulations

Let me tell you straight out: There are actually no regulations for the cosmetic and skincare industry. You or I could set up our own company today and start to sell our products without prior approval or authorization. Unlike with food products or drugs, the law does not require FDA approval for cosmetics and skincare products and their ingredients, other than color additives, before they go on the market.

According to the FDA website, "companies and individuals who manufacture or market cosmetics have a legal responsibility to ensure the safety of their products. Neither the law nor FDA regulations require specific tests to demonstrate the safety of individual products or ingredients. The law also does not require cosmetic companies to share their safety information with FDA." This means that the market for skincare products is a little like the Wild West, showing very little concern for consumer safety.

This lack of regulation is why fads appear and disappear with alarming regularity and leave us all open to unscrupulous operators who are more interested in our money than the health of our skin. Technically, everyone can make creams and sell them without many consequences if they don't live up to expectations.

Globally, there are trade federations and approval systems, but none are compulsory and barriers to entry to the skincare markets just don't exist.

All of this can leave you vulnerable to scams and fads and seriously out of pocket without making any improvement to your skin, and worse, damaging it.

No more wondering "what's her secret?" for beautiful skin

Growing up, I would hear my mom telling me, "Wow, I saw this lady who has such beautiful skin. I wonder what her secret is? She told me that she eats two raw tomatoes every day. I wonder if that's the reason for her beautiful skin?"

Throughout my years growing up and specializing in skincare, people have been sharing their secrets with me: They often recommend eating certain fruits, applying certain oils, or sticking to a specific diet.

Of course, when someone we know shares her "secret" with us, we want to try it because we want to look like that person. (Remember my story about the infomercial featuring the supermodel? It motivated me to almost purchase a product over the phone.)

However, having beautiful, healthy-looking skin is not a mystery. THERE IS NO SECRET! Once you know the basics of what the skin is and what causes aging skin, you will know how to prevent it from aging and even be able to reverse the signs of aging.

After reading this book, you will learn the function of the skin, the causes of aging skin, and when to use what for your skin. Your skin changes with time as you age, as the seasons change, and as the temperature changes. So, of course, your skin needs will change. Chapter 2 will teach you the basics about skin and signs of aging. Chapter 3 will show you how to prevent aging skin through lifestyle changes and by choosing products wisely and looking for the ingredients in skincare cream that will work for you. Chapter 4 is about the actions you can take to reverse the signs of aging. And finally, Chapter 5 will put it all together and describe a stepwise approach, so you know when to use what. Reading this book will take you a long way toward knowing what works best for your skin.

CHAPTER 2: THE BASICS OF SKIN AND THE CAUSES OF AGING SKIN

The functions of the skin

The first thing we need to learn is skin basics. The question is – what is the skin and what does it do? Although it is not often thought of in this way, your skin is the largest organ of the body. It is the thin layer of tissue that covers your body with a natural protective layer. Skin is the part of your body that first comes into contact with outside forces. Because of this, the skin performs some important functions that help the rest of the body to live.

Our skin is our armor, and because it gets exposed to external elements every day, we must protect it and make sure that it stays healthy so that it can protect us in return. Our skin helps us in many ways. It protects the rest of the body from microbes, physical damage and dehydration. The protective layer of the skin forms a waterproof mechanical layer that prevents microbes from entering our body, unless the skin is broken.

Another way the skin protects us from disease is by alerting the immune system to the presence of harmful organisms by producing and excreting antibacterial substances, and supporting the growth of "healthy" bacteria.

The skin is also a hugely important factor in keeping us alive by regulating our body temperature. We need to maintain a steady temperature of 98.6°F to be able to function normally. The body's normal core temperature is between 98°F and 100°F. When our body temperature goes a little off, we don't feel very well. When our temperature goes way off (too low or too high), we are in grave danger of death.

The skin reacts to the changes in outside temperature and internal factors to regulate body temperature. It opens up pores when we are hot. This allows you to sweat, permits heat to be released and cools your temperature back down to the 98.6° that our body needs to function normally.

When you are cold, the skin closes the pores, stops you from sweating and makes the hairs on your skin stand on end to prevent further heat loss.

The skin is the organ of the body that helps you to have the sensation of touch. This is a very important part of the way you interact with the world around you. As one of the five senses, touch helps you detect the dangers around you and react accordingly. The sensation of touch is transferred to the brain by sensory receptors in the skin. They allow you to feel pain, pressure and heat in the objects around you. This, in turn, gives you the chance to react in the appropriate way when you encounter something. When you encounter an object that causes you pain, your skin delivers this very useful information to the rest of your body and enables you to take evasive action and store this information so you don't make the same mistake again.

So to clarify, the functions of the skin are:

- **Protection against microbes**
- **Regulation of body temperature**
- **The defense that comes with the sense of touch**

The three layers of the skin

The skin is made up of three layers that all play their part in what makes your skin the useful and remarkable organ that helps you in your everyday life. The three layers of the skin are the epidermis, dermis and hypodermis. The epidermis is the thin layer of the skin that sits at the outermost part of the body, the protective layer that is constantly being replaced from the layers below it as we shed skin cells through the activities we carry out in everyday life.

The epidermis, your body's natural armor

The epidermis' properties allow it to repel water from the outside but also to retain the correct moisture levels inside the body. It can be seen as a membrane that can regulate water levels. The epidermis also determines your skin tone, and this is why it is an important consideration when it comes to skincare. Your skin tone will play a part in the ingredients you need when it comes to selecting and using your skin cream. The epidermis is also where Ultraviolet B (UVB) rays can help trigger the synthesis of vitamin D, which is an essential vitamin for your body functions.

The dermis, the "go-between"

The dermis is the largest layer of the skin and sits between the epidermis and the hypodermis. It is responsible for providing nutrients and physical support to the epidermis. Your dermis is made up of 90 percent collagen, making it the part of the skin that provides elasticity, strength and resistance.

As a protective barrier, your skin needs to be strong because it is the first line of defense for you when it comes to repelling outside forces. When skin is stretched, the collagen fibers prevent tearing as a result of their high tensile strength. The dermis is also filled with elastic fibers, so they can react to the things around you.

If you touch something with your finger, you will notice that, after the pressure is removed, your skin returns to its normal shape. It doesn't hold the point of pressure in it as an indentation. This is the elastic fibers doing their thing and making sure that your skin bounces back to its normal configuration. This is important because, once you lose these elastic fibers, sagging begins to occur. The dermis also contains blood vessels that carry nutrients to the epidermis to keep it alive and healthy.

The dermis also has nerve fibers that transmit the sensations of touch from your skin to your brain. This transmission from skin to brain is how the body transforms contact into a sensation. Your brain can then react to that sensation in the appropriate manner. If the sensation is pleasant, you may want to continue to experience it. If the sensation is unpleasant, you will want to stop it from happening by moving away.

The dermis contains hair follicles, sebaceous glands that secrete sebum, and sweat glands. They play an important role in helping your body regulate temperature. Sweat is especially important for temperature regulation; the ability to sweat gives your body the control it needs to help you survive in the environment you are in.

The sebum from the sebaceous gland has many wonderful functions, such as covering the surface of the hairs and protecting them from drying and becoming brittle, inhibiting excessive evaporation of water from skin so that skin remains soft and supple, acting as a skin lubricant, and having antifungal and antibacterial properties. Sebum's antifungal and antibacterial properties are due to its acidic nature, making it an unfavorable environment for many harmful microbes.

The hypodermis, "the inside fat guy"

The hypodermis is the skin layer that is innermost and, like the other two, performs important functions that help you go about your daily business. The hypodermis consists mainly of fat, so it helps your body insulate itself against the elements outside of the body that can affect temperature, for example, by keeping you warm on a cold day.

The tissues found in the hypodermis contain fat that is used as the body's energy reserve. During intense effort or when the body lacks energy, the fat found in the fat tissue can be put back into the blood circulation, via your veins (the venous route), and then transformed into energy. When we speak of "burning up calories", we mean that we are burning up fats in particular. The skin is the ideal place to store the energy because it is all over the body so can quickly deliver the energy needed on short notice.

The other key factor to know about the hypodermis is that it is made up of connective tissue. This is the tissue that connects the upper layers of the skin to the rest of the body.

What we've learned so far about the skin's structure and functions
In all, the skin performs many key functions of the body and helps to keep us alive and well. Your skin is a part of the body that covers all the other parts and as such is an important barrier that keeps you safe from impact and disease. Your skin needs to be in top condition to be able to help your body look after itself and perform all the necessary functions. You need to learn to protect your skin so that it can protect you.

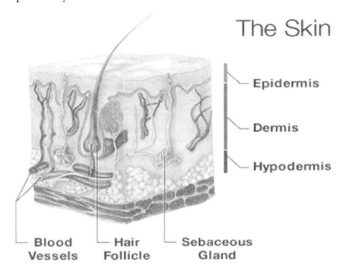

The Skin
- Epidermis
- Dermis
- Hypodermis
- Blood Vessels
- Hair Follicle
- Sebaceous Gland

Image from: http://www.dianesays.com/foods-and-habits-for-healthy-beautiful-skin/

The two ways skin ages
Now that you understand the basics of the skin, what it's made up of and how it functions, we can move on to understand the basic factors that cause skin to age. Before we can prevent or combat aging skin, we need to learn what causes it to age in the first place. The two ways skin ages are intrinsic and extrinsic.

Intrinsic aging of the skin

Intrinsic aging can be seen as the normal course of aging that happens to all of us as we get older. With age, our body changes and starts to deteriorate, so all these changes will affect our skin and its appearance. Internal factors that can cause aging skin are inflammation, hormonal imbalance, nutrient deficiency, and loss of cells.

Inflammation: One type of internal inflammation is caused by the level of cortisol in our bodies; cortisol is also known as the stress hormone. Elevated cortisol levels are caused when we feel stressed. In the short term, these elevated cortisol levels can be good for us, for example, when we need a burst of energy to flee danger.

However, if we are constantly stressed, the levels of cortisol that brings about can cause inflammation. This internal inflammation will lead to acne breakouts, rosacea and visible signs of aging, such as wrinkles and sagging, because inflammation increases the breakdown of collagen. Remember collagen plays an important role in our dermis layer to maintain the strength and suppleness of the skin. This means we do not want the loss of collagen.

Hormonal imbalance: Hormonal changes in your body can have a big effect on your skin and the way it looks and feels. There is a natural decrease in estrogen, progesterone, and testosterone as we get older and are heading towards menopause. These hormones have multiple functions in our body. But with respect to skin, the loss of estrogen will lead to increased dryness and wrinkling, as well as a decrease in collagen. As you get older, this means that the skin produces less collagen and elastin, which are the parts of your skin that give it both flexibility and the ability to stay taut. Loss of estrogen and the subsequent loss of collagen and elastin cause your skin to lose some of that ability to stay looking supple, smooth and young.

Nutrient deficiency: As we age, our body will produce less nutrients that are good for the skin. These nutrients include natural antioxidants, such as vitamin C, vitamin E, and Coenzyme Q10. These antioxidants help fight against the harmful effects of UV rays. The cells in our body are exposed to oxygen every day, which causes oxidation. In oxidation, body chemicals are altered and form free radicals (also called reactive oxygen species [ROS]). Over time, free radicals can cause a chain reaction in our body that damages important body chemicals, DNA and parts of our cells. Some cells can heal, while others are permanently damaged.

Scientists believe free radicals may contribute to the aging process, as well as cause diseases such as cancer, diabetes and heart disease. Antioxidants are natural substances that may stop or limit the damage caused by free radicals by stabilizing the free radicals. This keeps them from causing damage to other cells. Because our skin is constantly exposed to free radicals and oxidation, antioxidants play an important role in fighting the damage caused by free radicals.

With age also comes a decrease in essential fatty acids, which are important in keeping our skin moisturized. Without them, our skin will become very dry. Alpha-lipoic acid, another nutrient that decreases as we age, helps improve our immune system, neutralizes free radicals, protects collagen, and works together with other antioxidants. Last but not least is the decrease of hyaluronic acid. Hyaluronic acid is a large sugar molecule found in collagen-rich tissues. Its functions are to attract and bind water and provide volume and fullness, as well as maintain smoothness and moisture in the skin. Half of the hyaluronic acid in the human body is depleted by age 50 due to free radical damage. Most of this loss happens in the epidermis, and not so much in the dermis.

Loss of cells: As we age, the number of cells responsible for our skin tone decreases, and they have a tendency to cluster together. This creates the appearance of brown spots, also known as age spots.

Ethnicity: Ethnicity plays a large part in your skin's aging process. Darker skin is more resistant to the aging process and those with darker skin will see less of the signs of aging as they get older. For example, African Americans and Asians who have dark skin develop less wrinkles, and their wrinkles are less pronounced as they get older. The ethnicity you have plays a part in how quickly you age and how your skin looks as you get older.

Characteristics of intrinsic aging

As your skin goes through the process of intrinsic aging, certain signs of this process manifest themselves on your face. The inner layers of your skin shrink, causing the fibers to be less organized and the layers of the skin to be less tight. The effect is that your skin starts to sag a little and fine wrinkles occur. The fine wrinkles are the result of the breakdown of collagen levels and the first visible sign of aging most women want to deal with as they age.

These signs reflect the general loss of elasticity in the skin. You will notice that your skin no longer feels as elastic as it once did. In addition to this, the surface of your skin starts to feel rough. Intrinsic aging is part of the way the whole body ages and also a part of life. It cannot be avoided completely and is just the way your body reacts to the changes in age, loss of nutrients, and reduction in hormone levels.

Extrinsic aging of the skin

Extrinsic aging is the other effect on your skin and the way it looks and feels. Unlike intrinsic aging, extrinsic aging is caused by many external factors.

There are things that we do to our skin and that our skin experiences in daily life that can damage it and change the way it performs for us. You have control over the effects of these outside forces, so you can minimize those ill effects.

Here are some factors you need to be aware of when it comes to the extrinsic aging of your skin:

Extreme temperatures: Extreme temperatures change the way your skin reacts and performs because it has to work harder to regulate your temperature.

High temperatures increase water evaporation from your skin and can leave it feeling dehydrated. Water plays a very important part in all of the functions of the body and skin is no different. You need to keep your skin hydrated, so it can perform at its best and carry out all the vital tasks it is designed to carry out. If you lose water from your skin on a regular basis, you greatly increase your chances of having very visible signs of aging later in life.

Low temperatures, on the other hand, cause hardening and reduced water loss. Cold weather and harsh winds can cause the oils on our skin to go out of balance, making it extremely dry. The right balance of oils is important to keep the skin healthy and young-looking. This contributes in a big way to premature aging.

Repeated sun exposure (UV rays): Aside from the potential of skin cancer, which still kills more than 10,000 people every year in the USA alone, exposure to the sun increases your chances of prematurely aging skin. Up to 90 percent of the visible skin changes commonly attributed to aging are caused by the sun.

UV rays are a little dose of radiation that creates reactive oxygen species (ROS) that can damage DNA and lead to skin cancer; exposure to these rays breaks down the layers of the skin, especially collagen, which is very important to the integrity of our skin. It breaks down the skin in a way that produces sagging, opens pores and increases the number of wrinkles.

Constant exposure to UV rays not only causes premature aging of the skin but also signs of sun damage such as age spots, actinic keratosis (which is a scaly or crusty growth lesion), and solar elastosis (where skin appears yellow and thickened as a result of sun damage). All of these are signs of aging that we can avoid. Our skin turning red is a sign that we have damaged it and have contributed to the aging process. Multiply the occurrence of this skin-reddening by the number of times it happens, and you are looking at a lot of damage over a long period of time.

Pollution: Because of the many vehicles on our roads and heavy industry, pollutants are in the air everywhere, especially in big cities. In fact, you may find that pollutants are really difficult to avoid if you live or work in a city, but you need to be aware of the aging effect they have on your skin.

All the smog, dirt, dust, grime, car exhaust fumes and even the pesticides that are flying around in the air will get into your skin at some stage. As we have seen, your skin is a permeable layer, so, although it can keep out microbes, it cannot keep out everything that is in the air you breathe and live in.

Pollution consists of polycyclic aromatic hydrocarbons (PAHs), which are a group of more than 100 different chemicals released from oil, gasoline, burning coal, trash, tobacco, wood, or other substances, such as charcoal-broiled meat. Research has shown that these PAHs are bound to nanoparticles in the air and are converted to quinones. Quinones, in turn, produce reactive oxygen species (ROS), which result in the same type of skin aging we see with chronic exposure to UV light. Quinones not only prematurely age the skin through the creation of ROS, but they are also thought to cause skin pigmentation.

Cigarette smoking: Many studies have been carried out that describe the correlation between cigarette smoking and premature aging, and they have all come to the same conclusion – that smoking is bad for your skin.

Smoking actually has two ill effects on the skin. The first is that the nicotine in the cigarette restricts blood flow, which, in turn, restricts the body's ability to get vital oxygen and nutrients to the skin. This makes the skin less efficient, and the lack of nutrients contributes to the break-down in the layers of skin.

The second way cigarette smoking affects the skin is through the chemicals that are blown out of the mouth from a cigarette. These chemicals come in close contact with the skin and can cause premature aging in a similar manner to other pollutants.

Repetitive facial muscle movements, such as squinting, smiling or frowning: When you are young, as your skin moves, the elastic fibers in your body help it spring back into shape. But over time these fibers break down and, with repetitive motion, they can become less elastic, creating small and deep wrinkles. I would never recommend that you stop smiling. Don't worry: I will show you how to reverse those smile lines in Chapter 4. However, I do recommend that you try to squint and frown less.

Poor nutrition: The saying "you are what you eat" is definitely true when it comes to the signs of aging skin. Poor nutrition will show on your skin. The nutrients that we take in help to keep the skin healthy and looking great. Poor nutrition means that you won't get all of the right things your skin needs to keep it in top shape. As you get older this has a bigger impact on your fight against the signs of aging because your body is automatically losing nutrients already. A balanced diet with all the right nutrients will help keep your skin in the best shape it can be.

Lack of sleep: Lack of sleep is an external factor that affects the skin's ability to recuperate and recover overnight when you are asleep. Just as your body recovers during sleep, so too does your skin. You need to ensure that you get the right amount of sleep so that your skin can be ready for the next day. Without sleep, your body will release more cortisol and less human growth hormone, thus aging your skin prematurely.

Reduced water intake: Over time reduced water intake will cause dehydration and result in premature aging of the skin. This is because it has less and less of the water and nutrients it needs to perform its vital tasks. Dehydration will affect the balance of oils on your skin and its ability to regenerate. Your skin is one of the organs that depends on a constant supply of water to survive and thrive.

Alcohol consumption: The effect alcohol has on the appearance of your skin cannot be overstated.

You will notice yourself that, after a heavy night of alcohol consumption, your skin looks sallow and dehydrated. Alcohol can leave you dehydrated, causing your skin to look more wrinkly. Over time, repeated overconsumption of alcohol will damage your skin irreparably. And, as you get older, those negative effects multiply.

Stress: Stress pervades all aspects of life from home to work and everywhere in between. Although it can be difficult to manage, managing stress is worth it, given its impact on how quickly your skin ages.

As I have said elsewhere in this book, constant stress is not good for you because it increases your cortisol levels, which is bad for your skin. You want to eliminate stress as much as possible to avoid premature aging. Stress contributes to sleepless nights, with the resultant bags under your eyes.

Stress at work can cause you to take in fewer fluids, and we have seen the potential damage that can cause. Stress can also lead to increased alcohol intake and the negative effects to the body that brings with it.

In Chapter 3, I will go into detail about how to counteract these external factors that cause extrinsic aging.

What we've learned so far about the factors that influence intrinsic and extrinsic aging of the skin

As a result of all these extrinsic aging factors, your skin comes under attack daily from extreme temperatures, repeated sun exposure, pollution, smoking, repetitive movement of the facial muscles, poor nutrition, lack of sleep, alcohol consumption and stress And we saw the signs of intrinsic aging as being the shrinking of inner layers of the skin, skin surface roughness, fine wrinkles and a loss of elasticity. However, the signs of extrinsic aging are very different, as we will see in the next part of this book.

But before we look at the signs of extrinsic aging, **let me remind you about the good news**: You have control over the effects of extrinsic aging.

The characteristics of extrinsic aging

When you take a step back, you can see that the effects of intrinsic aging are of lesser severity and cannot be controlled, whereas the signs of extrinsic aging are more severe but, at the same time, can be controlled or managed by changes to your lifestyle. That is the way you need to look at the whole science behind the aging of your skin – especially the premature aging of your skin.

Deeper wrinkles show on your face much more easily than fine wrinkles and are a common sign of extrinsic aging. The skin creams on the market play to this by talking about deep wrinkles and the way their creams will deal with them. But I always think that prevention is a much better option than a cure.

Deep wrinkles are one of the main reasons people steer away from skin creams and toward more radical solutions. Botox and other injections are a popular way to smooth out the skin and create a wrinkle-free image to present to the world. However, we want to deal with the issue before it actually begins to happen and get ahead of the game.

Blotchy skin, which is patches of discolored skin, is another sign of extrinsic aging that can cause your skin to look older and appear to be in worse condition than it actually is. Women all over the world try to conceal blotchy skin with make-up. Blotchy skin is a general term that describes skin that doesn't look normal. Many things cause it. However, in terms of extrinsic aging, it is caused by UV rays from the sun.

Exposure to UV radiation causes an increase in melanin, a pigment responsible for our skin color, resulting in darker skin color. With repeated sun exposure, you will end up getting sun spots, those dark spots that dot your skin. People become embarrassed by blotchy skin and don't want others to see it. As a result, they will spend money on makeup to cover up the blemishes or on expensive creams that promise to get rid of them altogether.

So what if you could put a plan in place to look at all the factors that age your skin and start to eradicate them from your life as much as possible? Well, you can. But before we get to the plan, let's continue our skincare education.

Wrinkles – how do they occur?

Wrinkles are the number one way people notice that their face looks older. As we look in the mirror, we notice that we have developed these lines on our face that were not there when we were younger. The wrinkles are the driving force behind much of the skincare industry because consumers either want to get rid of the wrinkles they have or want to look after their skin in a way that stops wrinkles from ever forming. It also drives the other side of the industry that looks into procedures or surgery to get rid of wrinkles. As with much of this book, I recommend combatting wrinkles by actually knowing the basics about them. So what causes wrinkles?

Reduced muscle mass: As the muscles in your face start to atrophy naturally over time, they weaken or disappear in places. The lack of muscle mass behind the skin is one of the factors that causes the skin to appear less tight and wrinkles to develop in the areas where the muscles used to be. That is why you often hear people recommending different ways to stimulate your muscle mass, such as massage or facial exercises.

Reduced skin thickness: As the three layers of the skin – the epidermis, the dermis and the hypodermis – get thinner, they are less able to provide the barrier that your body requires. Reduced skin thickness causes wrinkles to appear and your skin to look older than it is. Maintaining skin thickness is one way to prevent wrinkles, and as you recall, the dermis is the thickest layer out of the three layers of the skin. To maintain a thicker skin layer, you need to maintain your dermis layer, which brings us to the next point…

Collagen and elastin loss, damage, or abnormal restructuring: Remember that your dermis is made up of 90 percent collagen; it is the part of the skin that provides elasticity, strength and resistance. As you get older, the amount of collagen in your skin will lessen, leading to stiffened collagen and a loss of normal skin structure. At the same time, the elastin fibers lose their elasticity over time, and that also causes skin to have abnormal structure. Together, these two effects result in the appearance of wrinkled skin.

Time is not the only thing that causes the loss of collagen and elastin. Extrinsic factors, such as smoking, poor diet, and UV radiation can damage collagen and elastin. With a less strong, less elastic and less resistant skin, wrinkles start to appear. We cannot turn back time, but we can find ways to prevent the loss, damage and breakdown of collagen and elastin, which, in turn, will prevent or reverse the signs of aging.

Dehydration of the skin: Remember that raisins are dehydrated grapes. The loss of water causes the grape to shrivel and have lots of wrinkles and turn into a raisin. This is what we will look like if we don't maintain hydration for our body. Some experts think that as many as 75 percent of the U.S. population suffers from dehydration.

We lose water from sweating, exposure to extremes in temperature, or illness. Also, as we get older, it becomes harder for water to enter our cells. Water is vital for our bodily functions, so when our body is dehydrated, priority will be given to our vital organs, such as the brain, lungs, and heart, for access to whatever water the body has on hand. Our skin is not a high priority in comparison to our vital organs, so the signs of dehydration will show first on our skin.

As a result of dehydration, our skin will become dry, flaky, and wrinkled. Skin may feel tight and have similar symptoms to those of sunburn; people will sometimes experience a burning sensation or extreme itching. Itching causes scratching, which can make skin painful or turn it red. This then leads to more skin damage and more wrinkles.

The bottom line: We have to keep our skin and body hydrated, preventing it from drying and shriveling up, making us look like a wrinkled raisin.

What we've learned so far about maintaining healthy skin
Up to this point in the book, we have learned the influence marketing has on our skincare choices and the basics of the skin and its functions. We also now understand the causes of intrinsic and extrinsic aging and how wrinkles occur. Armed with this knowledge, we can devise a plan to prevent skin from aging, and also reverse the aging process.

An overall plan for skin anti-aging
Prevention is always better than the cure, especially when it comes to the challenges of aging skin. It is so much easier to get your plan in place as early in life as you can and find the ways to look after your skin as best as possible all along the way, rather than having to back-peddle.

An important part of that plan is finding the products with all the right ingredients for you to have skin you can be proud of and that doesn't age prematurely. There are certain key steps you want to take on this path to healthy skin.

Prevention

1. Prevent or counteract the negative effects of intrinsic aging, to the extent that you can

To review what we have learned about the causes of intrinsic aging: The signs of our body's natural aging process are chronic inflammation, nutrient deficiency, hormonal change, and ethnicity.

Unfortunately, we cannot do much about our ethnicity and the decrease in our hormones and body's nutrients as we age. However, we can **counteract nutrient deficiency by eating right and using skincare creams that contain these nutrients**.

We can also **prevent chronic inflammation by trying to maintain a low level of cortisol** (also known as the stress hormone). I know it is easier said than done, especially the older we get, but it is a fact that the more stress we have, the more it shows on our face. We can **counter the inflammatory effects of cortisol by eating food and using dietary supplements that are known to be anti-inflammatory**. We can adopt practices to lessen stress, such as meditation and mindfulness, as well as exercise. In addition, we also need to use skincare creams that contain the nutrients that are good for our skin.

2. Prevent the negative effects of extrinsic aging by changing your lifestyle

As we have learned, extrinsic aging is due to external factors, and it is easier to prevent their negative effects on our skin by changing our lifestyle. The external factors we talked about are **extreme temperature, UV radiation, pollution, cigarette smoking, and repetitive facial muscle movements such as frowning, poor nutrition, lack of sleep, reduced water intake, alcohol, and stress.**

We want to avoid exposing our skin to temperatures that are too hot or too cold. Avoiding UV radiation is very important to prevent premature skin aging because UV rays damage the collagen and elastin. Therefore, we need to protect our skin from the sun and tanning beds. Pollution and cigarette smoking are bad for your skin, so try to avoid exposing your skin to both as much as possible.

Try to eat healthy, get plenty of sleep, increase water intake, and decrease alcohol consumption, as well as your stress level. One thing that's hard to avoid is repetitive facial muscle movements. I wouldn't tell you to stop smiling. But you can try to avoid frowning or squinting. And to help, I will discuss in detail how to combat wrinkles and lessen their degree in Chapter 4.

3. Prevent wrinkles from forming

Because wrinkles are the main sign of aging, we want to prevent their formation. We just learned that wrinkles occur due to the loss of muscle mass, skin thinning, loss of collagen and elastin, as well as dehydration. So in order to prevent the development of wrinkles, we need to prevent the loss of muscle mass and the thinning of the skin by maintaining the integrity of the skin's collagen and elastin. We also need to maintain hydration for our body and our skin so that our skin is hydrated and won't become dry and wrinkly.

You have seen the factors that can cause wrinkles and the signs of aging in the skin. Your dream is to have skin without wrinkles and blemishes through prevention. The plan that you put together and the way you stick to this plan will help you greatly with seeing that dream become a reality. You can have an effect on the way that your skin looks. You can be the master of your own destiny and make some simple, but effective, lifestyle changes that will help you and your skin look better.

Just by changing a few things in your life, you will give yourself your best chance of producing your own natural anti-aging solutions without the need for solutions out of a bottle, from a needle or under the knife. Your plan should be all about taking control of the situation yourself and doing something positive for the health and look of your skin.

Treatment

Depending on when you started your prevention plan, how well you have stuck to it and what stage of life you have now reached, you will get to the point where some wrinkles start to appear. The fine wrinkles that are a natural part of the aging process are nothing to be unduly worried about, but when wrinkles appear, you want to know ahead of time what you can do to deal with them.

The way you prevent wrinkles from happening is through lifestyle changes that you are able to make and by implementing a consistent plan over a number of years. The results can be seen in the way your face does not age prematurely. The changes you make today will have positive effects on the way your skin looks in a year's time, five years' time, ten years' time, or twenty years' time and beyond. But what can you do if wrinkles are staring you in the face every time you look in the mirror now?

What are the solutions to treating wrinkles as opposed to trying to prevent them from happening? As I mentioned earlier, we cannot completely prevent the formation of wrinkles. Intrinsic factors such as changes in hormone levels, our ethnicity, and repetitive facial muscle movements are a few things that are unavoidable. Therefore, we need to prepare ourselves ahead of time to know the steps we will take to combat the wrinkles that do develop so that we can reverse the fine lines or decrease the severity of the wrinkles. We also need to know how we can reverse the other signs of aging, such as the blotchy dark spots caused by the sun or advancing age.

I still maintain that prevention is better than the cure, but there are ways to help your skin fight back against wrinkles and blotchy discolored skin.

1. Implement solutions to address the intrinsic effects of aging
To help fight back against the wrinkles you have now, you can try to reverse intrinsic aging by using hormone replacement therapy, nutrient supplements, and anti-inflammatory remedies. With respect to hormone replacement therapy, the goal is to supplement your body with bio-identical hormones to get it back to a normal level. This method is not for everyone, so you need to consult with your healthcare provider first before you do this.

Because our body makes fewer of the nutrients that are good for our skin as we age and because inflammation causes skin to age, we can take actions to counteract the ill effects of both of these things. We can eat foods containing the nutrients our skin needs and that are known to be anti-inflammatory. We can choose supplements that have anti-inflammatory effects and that contain those vital nutrients, and we can use skin creams with the necessary nutrients and anti-inflammatory ingredients.

2. Avoid the extrinsic forces that affect skin negatively

Also, to reverse the signs of aging, you still need to avoid the extrinsic factors that I mentioned in the prevention section of this book. If you are a smoker, this is a great time to stop smoking completely and give your skin the best chance of holding on to the collagen that it already has. You need the collagen in the dermis layer of your skin to keep your skin strong and resistant.

Avoiding extreme temperatures, UV radiation, and pollution, as well as eating healthy foods, getting adequate sleep in addition to increasing water intake, decreasing alcohol consumption and stress are all things you can do to stop and maybe even reverse the aging process.

The skin is wonderful because it constantly regenerates. New skin cells are constantly forming, so stopping the bad habits and allowing the skin time to heal will pay off as the skin renews itself.

3. Reverse wrinkling, especially deep wrinkles

Ways to reverse wrinkling are to increase muscle mass, reduce collagen breakdown while stimulating its production, prevent further skin-thinning, increase skin smoothness, and increase hydration and water retention of the skin. We will go into more detail about this in Chapter 4 of this book.

The fact that you are monitoring your skin closely is a good thing. It is the first step to getting a plan together to deal with it. Awareness is crucial. From here you need to consider the things that are important when it comes to getting your skin back in shape as soon as possible.

This is what we will be looking at in the last part of this book. Treating your skin at this time is the best way to take back control and put you and your skin on the right track for you. Remember the key areas that we have discussed and make the changes that will promote healthy skin and get control back over those wrinkles.

CHAPTER 3: HOW TO PREVENT WRINKLES FROM HAPPENING

We have come a long way together, and there is still some way to go. But to move forward, it is often the best course of action to pause and take a little look back. We have looked at the skin and the way it functions. Now we know what the skin is made up of, so we can see what we can do to help protect it. Once we know the building blocks of the skin, we can implement changes to our diet and lifestyle that will help us have better skin – not just for now but for the rest of our life.

We then looked at the two different types of aging. Intrinsic aging is part of the body changing as you get older. It will happen naturally and is almost impossible to slow down or change. Aging that happens as a result of external influences on your skin is called "extrinsic". This type of aging is the one you have the most control over with the lifestyle choices you make.

Now that we know about our skin's makeup and functions, we need to look in more detail at how to protect it and prevent it from aging prematurely. You can do several things that will have a very big impact on the way your skin performs and ages.

The things you can do here are important, so consider changing the way you treat your skin starting today. You want to look and feel your best, so the steps you take to get there are important. Once you know the actions that you should be taking to look after your skin, you will be heading in the right direction. We have discussed all the different factors that can

affect your skin, so it makes sense to look at the key measures
you can take to counter these harmful factors.

Lifestyle changes

The things I will discuss in this part of the book are the
easiest steps you can take right now to make the biggest
difference in your skin and the way it looks – now and in the
future. These are things you can do on your own and turn
into habits that you will practice for the rest of your life.

Avoid extreme temperatures

Extreme temperatures could be due to natural causes, such as
heat waves, unseasonably cold weather, and winter storms.
They can also be due to manmade events, such as inadequate
home heating or cooling or extended exposure to
temperature extremes without proper gear. Try to minimize
the time you or your skin spend in these extreme
temperatures. If you cannot avoid the heat or cold, make sure
you wear proper gear to protect yourself. In extreme heat,
make sure you drink plenty of water to offset the water loss.
In extreme cold, use moisturizers to prevent your skin from
drying and wear enough clothes to keep yourself warm.

Avoid UV radiation

We already went over the negative effects of UV radiation,
how it can cause skin cancer and aging. There is UV radiation
caused by the sun, but there are also man-made UV rays that
we need to avoid. Examples of man-made UV radiation are
sunlamps and sunbeds (tanning beds and booths),
phototherapy (UV therapy), black-light lamps, mercury-vapor
lamps, and high-pressure xenon and xenon-mercury arc
lamps, plasma torches, and welding arcs.

People think that, just because these forms of radiation are indoors, they are safe. However, these man-made UV rays are just as harmful as the sun's UV radiation. According to skincancer.org, "a tan, whether you get it on the beach, in a bed, or through incidental exposure, is bad news, any way you acquire it. Tans are caused by harmful ultraviolet (UV) radiation from the sun or tanning lamps, and if you have one, you've sustained skin cell damage. No matter what you may hear at tanning salons, the cumulative damage caused by UV radiation can lead to premature skin aging (wrinkles, lax skin, brown spots, and more), as well as skin cancer. In fact, people who first use a tanning bed before age 35 increase their risk for melanoma by 75 percent."

In addition to avoiding man-made UV radiation, we need to avoid being outdoors in direct sunlight for too long. This is particularly important between the hours of 10 a.m. and 4 p.m. when UV light is strongest.

There's a shadow test that you can use to see how strong the sun's rays are. If your shadow is shorter than you are, the sun's rays are the strongest. There's also the UV Index, which is developed by the National Weather Service and the Environmental Protection Agency (EPA); the index gives people an idea of how strong the UV light is in their area every day, on a scale from 1 to 11+. A higher number means greater risk of exposure to UV rays and a higher chance of sunburn and skin damage that could ultimately lead to skin cancer. In the U.S., you can find your region's UV Index by going on the EPA's website (www.epa.gov/sunwise/uvindex.html) or downloading their mobile app through www.epa.gov/enviro/mobile.

According to cancer.org:

"UV rays reach the ground all year, even on cloudy or hazy days, but the strength of UV rays can change based on the time of year and other factors. UV rays become more intense in the spring, even before temperatures get warmer. People in some areas may get sunburned when the weather is still cool because they may not think about protecting themselves if it's not hot out.

"Be especially careful on the beach or in areas with snow because sand, water, and snow reflect sunlight, increasing the amount of UV radiation you get. UV rays can also reach below the water's surface, so you can still get a burn even if you're in the water and feeling cool. Some UV rays can also pass through windows. Typical car, home, and office windows block most UVB rays but a smaller portion of UVA rays, so even if you don't feel you're getting burned your skin may still get some damage. Tinted windows help block more UVA rays, but this depends on the type of tinting. (If you do have your car windows tinted, check local laws, as some states regulate this.) UV radiation that comes through windows probably doesn't pose a great risk to most people unless they spend long periods of time close to a window that gets direct sunlight."

If you must be outside, protect your skin with clothing: long-sleeved shirts, long pants and skirts cover the most skin and are the most protective. However, covering up doesn't block out all UV rays. UV rays can get through see-through fabric. Dark colors generally provide more protection than light colors. Tightly woven fabric protects better than loosely woven. Dry fabric is generally more protective than wet.

There are clothes that have a label listing the UV protection factor (UPF) value. The UPF value is the level of protection the garment provides from the sun's UV rays, on a range from 15 to 50+. The higher the UPF, the higher the protection from UV rays. These fabrics tend to be lightweight, tightly woven, and have special coatings to help absorb UV rays.

Now, clothing manufacturers offer new products that are used like laundry detergents in a washing machine. What's useful about these products is that they can increase the UPF value of clothes you already own. They add a layer of UV protection to your clothes without changing their color or texture. However, it's not exactly clear how much UV protection you get from using them.

In addition to wearing protective clothing, you need to use sunscreen. I will go into more detail about sunscreen later in this chapter. The other thing to wear is a broad-brimmed hat. "A hat with at least a 2- to 3-inch brim all around is ideal because it protects areas that are often exposed to intense sun, such as the ears, eyes, forehead, nose, and scalp. A dark, non-reflective underside to the brim can also help lower the amount of UV rays reaching the face from reflective surfaces such as water.

"A shade cap (which looks like a baseball cap with about 7 inches of fabric draping down the sides and back) is also good and will provide more protection for the neck. These shade caps are often sold in sports and outdoor supply stores. If you don't have a shade cap (or another good hat) available, you can make one by wearing a large handkerchief or bandana under a baseball cap. A baseball cap protects the front and top of the head but not the neck or the ears, where skin cancers commonly develop. Also, straw hats are not as protective as hats made of tightly woven fabric," according to cancer.org.

In Australia, an epidemic of skin cancer diagnoses in the 1980s and 1990s sparked a public awareness campaign devised by the government. That campaign went like this: "slip, slop, and slap." This stood for slip on a shirt, slop on the sunscreen and slap on a hat. It changed the public's perception of the sun and vastly reduced the incidences of skin cancer in the country over the years to the present day. The campaign is still used now.

We also need to wear sunglasses that block UV rays in order to protect our eyes and the delicate skin around our eyes. Extensive exposure of our eyes to sun without protection can increase our chances of developing cataracts or cancer. You need to buy sunglasses that block 99 to 100 percent of UVA and UVB rays. Before you buy, check the label to make sure the sunglasses you're buying have this kind of protection. Labels that say "UV absorption up to 400 nm" or "Meets ANSI UV Requirements" mean the glasses block at least 99 percent of UV rays. Those labeled "cosmetic" block about 70 percent. Don't assume the sunglasses provide any UV protection if there is no label.

Glasses that are darker are not necessarily better because UV protection comes from an invisible chemical in or applied to the lenses, not from the color or darkness of the lenses. Look for an ANSI label. Try to use large-framed and wrap-around sunglasses because they can protect your eyes from light coming in from different angles. Children need smaller versions of protective adult sunglasses. You should not buy your children toy sunglasses.

As I mentioned in Chapter 2, vitamin D is made by exposing unprotected skin to sunlight. Vitamin D has a lot of health benefits, including lowering the risk of some cancers, as well as helping the absorption of calcium into our body. Currently, doctors are not sure what the optimal level of vitamin D is. Therefore, the current recommendation is to get vitamin D from your diet or vitamin supplements rather than from the sunlight because your diet and vitamin supplements do not increase the risk of skin cancer.

Avoid pollution

If you happen to live in a polluted environment, you can do several things to counter the effects of pollution on your skin. First, find out your daily air pollution forecasts in your area by downloading the State of the Air app put out by the American Lung Association on your mobile device or check the Air Quality Index from the EPA website. Try not to go out when air quality is bad. Always avoid exercising or going near high-traffic areas even when air quality is good because the vehicles on busy highways can create high pollution levels that can affect you up to one-third mile away.

If you need to go out when there's poor air quality, you need to wear protective garments to keep your skin from being exposed to pollution as much as possible. This includes clothing, hat, sunglasses, as well as a surgical face mask if you don't mind people looking at you funny. If you are one of those people who don't want to wear face masks, you need to clean your face thoroughly after you get home to remove the dirt, oil and debris from your pores.

Because pollution causes the production of free radicals that can damage your skin, you need to use antioxidants to counter these free radicals. I will discuss in detail about antioxidants later in this chapter. Other methods to avoid pollution include staying away from high-traffic areas during rush hour and using a good moisturizer that will create a barrier between your skin and pollution.

Quit cigarette smoking

To quit smoking is one of the best ways to keep your skin from aging prematurely. The pollutants from the cigarette smoke are very harmful to the skin. Smoking is one of the habits that not only affects you but also those around you, including your loved ones. You can speak to your doctor about the different ways to quit smoking, and many products and support services are available to help you quit smoking.

If someone you know smokes and you do not want to be exposed to second-hand smoke, encourage the person to quit. Do not allow that person to smoke in the house or in the car. Avoid the cigarette smoke as much as possible. Do not go into facilities that allow smoking. If you have to be in a facility that allows smoking (an example would be casinos), make sure you use the methods I discuss in the pollution section previously in this book: clean and exfoliate your skin thoroughly, use antioxidants and a good moisturizer.

Maintain good nutrition

As I mentioned in the section on intrinsic aging, our body will produce less nutrients as we age, and the chronic inflammation will lead to aging skin. Therefore, we should eat food that supplement the nutrients that are anti-inflammatory and good for our skin. To do this, you should consume foods that contain antioxidants and/or anti-inflammatory agents.

One of the most important nutrients for our skin is antioxidants. Although our body produces antioxidants to help fight free radicals formed through oxidation, we can get antioxidants by eating a healthy diet. We should eat food that contains antioxidants. Examples of antioxidants are vitamins A, C, and E, beta-carotene, lutein, lycopene, and selenium.

You would want to eat a diet that is a mixture of fruits and vegetables that contain a variety of antioxidants. You do not want to eat only one type of antioxidant, and moderation is key. Take a look at this table to see which foods contain which antioxidants.

Antioxidants	Examples of food containing the specified antioxidant
Vitamin A	Milk, liver, butter, eggs
Vitamin C	Found in most fruits and vegetables. Those with the highest amounts of vitamin C include papayas, strawberries, oranges, cantaloupe and kiwi, as well as bell peppers, broccoli, Brussels sprouts, tomatoes, cauliflower and kale.
Vitamin E	Found in some nuts and seeds, including almonds, sunflower seeds, hazelnuts and peanuts. It can also be found in green leafy vegetables, such as spinach and kale, and in oils, such as soybean, sunflower, corn and

	canola oils.
Beta-carotene	Found in colorful fruits and vegetables, including carrots, peas, cantaloupe, apricots, papayas, mangoes, peaches, pumpkin, apricots, broccoli, sweet potatoes and squash. It can also be found in some leafy green vegetables, including beet greens, spinach and kale.
Lutein	Found in green leafy vegetables, such as spinach, collards and kale, broccoli, corn, peas, papayas and oranges.
Lycopene	Found in pink and red fruits and vegetables, such as pink grapefruit, watermelon, apricots and tomatoes.
Selenium	Found in cereals (corn, wheat and rice), nuts, legumes, animal products (beef, fish, turkey, chicken, eggs and cheese), bread and pasta.

Some people choose to take antioxidant supplements. You should talk to your doctor if you are considering adding a supplement to your diet.

According to familydoctor.org:

"Many supplements do not contain a balance of vitamins, minerals and enzymes and can actually have a negative effect on your health. While foods that are rich in vitamin E and beta-carotene are very healthy and help reduce cancer risk, the U.S. Preventive Services Task Force and the American Academy of Family Physicians recommend against taking vitamin E or beta-carotene supplements for the prevention of cancer.

"People who smoke or have a high risk for lung cancer should not take supplemental beta-carotene because it can increase the risk of lung cancer. The best way to get antioxidants is by eating a diet with lots of vegetables, fruits, whole grains, seeds and nuts. Variety is also important. If you take a multi-vitamin supplement, be careful. Too much of some nutrients from supplements other than foods, such as vitamins E and A, or selenium, can be harmful. Be sure to talk to your doctor before taking any vitamin supplements."

Other types of food good for our skin are those that have an anti-inflammatory effect. This is because chronic inflammation is harmful to our body and will show on our skin.

Before we go into which foods are anti-inflammatory, we should look at the ones that promote inflammation so that we can avoid them. These are **refined carbohydrates**, such as white bread and pastries, **French fries** and other fried foods, **soda** and other sugar-sweetened beverages, **red meat** (burgers, steaks) and processed meat (hot dogs, sausage), **margarine**, shortening, and lard. These foods will promote inflammation and are bad for our health.

On the other hand, foods that are anti-inflammatory are foods that help calm our body's inflammation. The key anti-inflammatory players are omega-3 fatty acids, catechins, and curcumin. This is not a comprehensive list, but foods that

contain any of these ingredients will decrease the
inflammation in your body.

Anti-inflammatory ingredients	Examples of food
Omega-3 Fatty Acids	These contain high amounts of omega-3 fatty acids: flaxseed oil, flaxseed, fish oil, salmon, chia seeds.
Catechins	These contain high amounts of catechins: green tea, black tea, red wine (limit to 1 to 2 glasses a day), blackberries.
Curcumin	Turmeric, curry powder, and mango ginger.
Other foods that are anti-inflammatory	Olive oil, tomatoes, green leafy vegetables (spinach, kale, and collards), nuts (almonds and walnuts), fruits (strawberries, blueberries, cherries, and oranges), and fatty fish (mackerel, tuna, and sardines).

Good nutrition is the best prevention method for your health
and your skin. You can get a lot of the needed nutrients by
eating the right food.

These recommendations are not meant to overwhelm you,
but to help you in picking the right food for your skin and
health. One tip that I personally find useful is to blend a lot
of fruits and vegetables into a drink and take it every day. I

choose from the list of ingredients in this table, blend them together, split them up into single serving containers, and then store them in the freezer to be consumed later. This will save you time and still give you a lot of nutrients your body needs.

Get adequate sleep

Lack of sleep will cause your body to have an increase in cortisol levels, which is bad for your skin. But how much sleep is enough? Sleep needs vary from person to person. I myself cannot function without at least 7 to 8 hours of sleep a night while my husband only needs 6 to 7.

How much you sleep also depends on how old you are. Newborns sleep between 16 and 18 hours a day and children in preschool between 11 and 12 hours a day. School-aged children and adolescents need at least 10 hours of sleep each night.

As one gets older, the quality and quantity of sleep decreases.

According to "Your Guide to Healthy Sleep" published by **the National Institute of Health**:

"Despite variations in sleep quantity and quality, both related to age and between individuals, studies suggest that the optimal amount of sleep needed to perform adequately, avoid a sleep debt, and not have problem sleepiness during the day is about 7 – 8 hours for adults and at least 10 hours for school-aged children and adolescents. Similar amounts seem to be necessary to avoid an increased risk of developing obesity, diabetes, or cardiovascular diseases.

"Quality of sleep and the timing of sleep are as important as quantity. People whose sleep is frequently interrupted or cut short may not get enough of both non-REM sleep and REM sleep. Both types of sleep appear to be crucial for learning and memory—and perhaps for the restorative benefits of healthy sleep, including the growth and repair of cells."

Increase water intake

Hydration is crucial for our skin to stay young and healthy, so water intake needs to be sufficient for our body's needs. Water makes up 60 percent of our body weight, and it is vital for our survival. The important question is how much water you should drink each day to avoid dehydration. There is no easy answer because it depends on many factors, including your health, how active you are and where you live. An average, healthy adult living in a temperate climate requires about 13 cups (3 liters) of total beverages a day for men, and 9 cups (2.2 liters) for women, according to The Institute of Medicine.

We all heard the advice to drink eight 8-oz. glasses of water a day, so that's roughly about 1.9L. Although no hard evidence supports this advice, it's still popular because it's easy to remember. Healthy adults need 9 to 13 total cups **of beverages** a day; this includes water, food, and other beverages consumed throughout a day.

Food provides 20 percent of the daily water intake required because some food contains a lot of water. The "8 by 8" rule is still good to keep in mind. Make sure you adjust your water intake, depending on your environment and whether you exercise rigorously, as well as your health condition, and whether you are breastfeeding/pregnant or not.

One way to know that you are adequately hydrated is if you rarely feel thirsty or not. You can also check your urine color. If your urine is colorless or light yellow, you are adequately hydrated. To ensure that you drink enough water, drink a glass of water or other calorie-free or low-calorie beverage with each meal and between each meal, and drink water before, during and after exercise.

Decrease alcohol intake

Most of us drink alcohol occasionally. For many people, moderate drinking is probably safe although some people should not drink at all, including alcoholics, children, pregnant women, people taking certain medicines, and people with certain medical conditions. If you have questions about whether it is safe for you to drink, speak with your health care provider.

However, "safe" doesn't mean that it's good for you. Alcohol can leave you dehydrated, causing your skin to look more wrinkly. Drinking too much alcohol can increase your risk of high blood pressure, high triglycerides, liver damage, obesity, certain types of cancer, accidents and other problems. Red wine has been touted as the wine of choice because it contains resveratrol, an antioxidant, which may help prevent heart disease by increasing levels of high-density lipoprotein (HDL) cholesterol (the "good" cholesterol) and protecting against artery damage.

According to the Mayo Clinic:

"The resveratrol in red wine comes from the skin of grapes used to make wine. Because red wine is fermented with grape skins longer than is white wine, red wine contains more resveratrol. Simply eating grapes, or drinking grape juice, has been suggested as one way to get resveratrol without drinking alcohol. Red and purple grape juices may have some of the same heart-healthy benefits of red wine.

"Other foods that contain some resveratrol include peanuts, blueberries and cranberries. It's not yet known how beneficial eating grapes or other foods might be compared with drinking red wine when it comes to promoting heart health. The amount of resveratrol in food and red wine can vary widely. Resveratrol supplements also are available. While researchers haven't found any harm in taking resveratrol supplements, most of the resveratrol in the supplements can't be absorbed by your body."

I don't recommend that you start drinking red wine just because it contains resveratrol. After all, as we have just read, you can get this antioxidant from other foods as well. As I mentioned in the good nutrition section, there are many antioxidants available that you can consume, so don't set your heart on just one antioxidant, and don't start drinking alcohol because of it!

However, if you already drink red wine, do so in moderation. For healthy adults, that means up to one drink a day for women of all ages and men older than age 65, and up to two drinks a day for men age 65 and younger. The limit for men is higher because men generally weigh more and have more of an enzyme that metabolizes alcohol than women do. A drink is defined as 12 ounces (355 milliliters, or mL) of beer, 5 ounces (148 mL) of wine or 1.5 ounces (44 mL) of 80-proof distilled spirits.

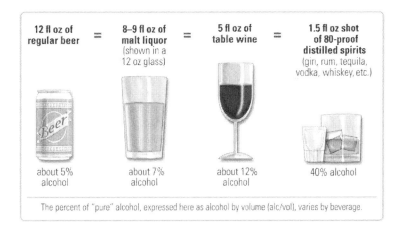

12 fl oz of regular beer	8–9 fl oz of malt liquor (shown in a 12 oz glass)	5 fl oz of table wine	1.5 fl oz shot of 80-proof distilled spirits (gin, rum, tequila, vodka, whiskey, etc.)
about 5% alcohol	about 7% alcohol	about 12% alcohol	40% alcohol

The percent of "pure" alcohol, expressed here as alcohol by volume (alc/vol), varies by beverage.

Image from: https://www.niaaa.nih.gov/alcohol-health/overview-alcohol-consumption/what-standard-drink

Decrease stress, and thus, cortisol levels

Stress and cortisol levels are correlated. The more stress you have, the more cortisol you have in your body, and this will increase inflammation in your body, resulting in premature skin aging.

To help decrease the amount of cortisol in your body, you can do some or all of the following: meditation, listening to your favorite music when you feel stress, getting adequate sleep, drinking some black tea, laughing more or hanging out with someone who makes you laugh, getting a massage, or exercising. All these activities have been shown to decrease cortisol levels and increase your "happy hormones" (dopamine and serotonin).

The bottom line: You want to do things that make you happy, relaxed, or both!

Products used to prevent aging skin

Remember when we looked at the ways people choose their skincare products? Well the fact that a celebrity is paid to promote a skin cream doesn't tell you whether it will help you. What you need to do is dig a little deeper and see the ingredients and protectors that you need and determine whether the products on the shelf will provide you with what you need. In this next part of the book, we will look at the types of products and ingredients you need to look for that will help protect your skin and prevent skin from aging. We will be discussing sunscreen, moisturizers, cleansers, lip balms, and ingredients that are antioxidants that can be found in skincare creams.

Sunscreen

One of the main extrinsic causes of skin damage is the harmful UV rays from the sun. So any plan that will be successful needs to consider this as a priority. What you need to do is make sure you prevent UV radiation from damaging the collagen and elastin.

The collagen and elastin in your skin provide it with the elastic and resistant qualities that are the opposite of wrinkled skin. A healthy young skin that is filled with collagen and elastin (like that of a baby) is always smooth and wrinkle-free. The UV rays will break these substances down, so the first step on the road to preventing skin from aging is protection from the sun.

The ideal way to be protected is to never encounter the sun again. But, of course, this is not practical. I already discussed the lifestyle choices you can make to protect yourself from the sun at the beginning of this chapter. A simple white T-shirt will provide an SPF factor of around 15, so it is not enough on its own to protect you from particularly strong UV rays.

You need to use a suitable level of sunscreen to keep your skin fully protected from the damage that the sun can do. Before we discuss the different types of sunscreens and how they protect us from UV radiation, we need to understand UV rays in detail.

Scientists often divide UV radiation into 3 wavelength ranges. These wavelengths are classified as UVA, UVB, and UVC, with UVA the longest of the three at 320 to 400 nanometers. UVA is further divided into two wave ranges, UVA 1, which measures 340 to 400 nanometers, and UVA 2, which extends from 320 to 340 nanometers. UVB ranges from 290 to 320 nm. UVC has the shortest wavelength ranges (100 to 290 nanometers), so most of it is absorbed by the ozone layer and does not reach the earth.

UV Ray	Wavelength
UVA1	340 - 400 nm
UVA2	320 - 340 nm
UVB	290 - 320 nm
UVC	110 - 290 nm

According to skincancer.org:

"Both UVA and UVB…penetrate the atmosphere and play an important role in conditions such as premature skin aging, eye damage (including cataracts), and skin cancers. They also suppress the immune system, reducing your ability to fight off these and other maladies."

UVA

UVA rays account for approximately 95 percent of the UV radiation that reaches the earth's surface from the sun. They are the prominent rays emitted by the sun. They are much less intense than the other types of UV rays we will look at shortly. UVA rays can penetrate clouds and glass, so their effects can be felt on the skin even on a cloudy day or while you are sitting near a window. You need to be aware of this all the time, so you can take appropriate steps to protect yourself. Don't think that because it is a cloudy day or that you are behind glass that you are 100 percent protected from the effects of UVA rays.

UVA rays, with their longer wavelength, penetrate deep into the dermis, where collagen and elastin are. Therefore, UVA rays are responsible for much of the damage we associate with photo-aging. Because UVA rays can reach the dermis, they damage the collagen fibers. This damage, in turn, causes increased production of abnormal elastin.

The unusual amounts of elastin result in the production of enzymes called metalloproteinases. These enzymes, which rebuild damaged collagen, often malfunction and degrade the collagen, resulting in incorrectly rebuilt skin. With repeated daily UVA exposure, the incorrectly rebuilt skin forms wrinkles, and the depleted collagen results in leathery skin. Recently, UVA exposure is also thought to contribute to skin cancer because the rays can damage the DNA in the cells in the epidermis as well.

UVB

Another type of UV ray is known as the UVB ray. UVB rays have slightly more energy than UVA rays. They can damage the DNA in skin cells directly, so they play a key role in the development of skin cancer and are thought to cause most skin cancers. They are also the main cause of sunburn and skin reddening, so they help contribute to skin tanning and photo-aging. They make up the other 5 percent of the UV radiation from the sun that reaches the surface of the earth.

UVB rays do not significantly penetrate glass, so you can find more protection from them while indoors, even if you are sitting next to a window. Unlike UVA, UVB rays only penetrate the epidermis, and not the dermis, so they are not the main cause for leathery-looking skin because they don't damage the collagen and elastin network.

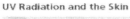

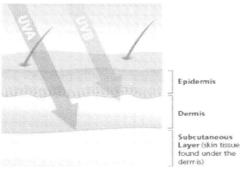

Image from: http://www.skincancer.org/prevention/uva-and-uvb

The different rays are classified by the wavelength at which they reach the earth. All three types of rays (UVA 1, UVA 2 and UVB) have wavelengths shorter than visible light, which means that they are invisible. If they were visible, the human race might have taken preventive action far sooner, in my view.

The fact that these rays are invisible means that the only visible sign that they have reached your skin is the redness and peeling that comes with sunburn – after the damage and potential cancerous effects have occurred.

Both UVA and the UVB rays will penetrate the atmosphere of the planet. This means that they play an important role in the conditions we are looking at in this book. But they can also cause eye damage, including the formation of cataracts and skin cancers for those who go unprotected. UVA and UVB rays also repress the immune system of the body. This results in a reduced ability to fight off the conditions we are discussing, as well as illnesses. Suffice it to say, the rays from the sun can be very harmful to the body in general and very harmful to the skin in particular.

UVC
The UVC rays emitted by the sun, as you might expect, are shorter than the others we've been discussing. UVC rays have more energy than the other types of UV rays, but luckily, they react with the ozone layer of the earth and never reach the atmosphere and are not a risk factor for skin cancer.

That is why the protection of the ozone layer is so important to the planet and the people who live on it. However, despite the protection the ozone layer offers from the sun's UVC rays, we find that man-made UVC radiation is still a concern. Man-made UVC radiation comes from arc welding torches, mercury lamps, and UV sanitizing bulbs that kill bacteria and other germs (such as in water, air, food, or on surfaces).

What to look for in sunscreen

Now that you know more about the damage caused by UV rays, you will want to use proper sunscreen to protect yourself from UVA and UVB radiation. Let's discuss some of the things you want to look for when you purchase sunscreen.

Broad Spectrum Sunscreen: Choose products that say "broad spectrum sunscreen". This means that the sunscreen can protect you from the sun's harmful UVA and UVB rays.

SPF 30 or higher: SPF stands for sunburn protection factor. It represents how well a sunscreen protects you from sunburn. A confusing thing about SPF is the number that follows it. This number tells you how much UVB light (the burning rays) a sunscreen can filter out. The SPF number does not have anything to do with UVA protection. **SPF 15** means 93 percent of the sun's UVB rays are filtered out. **SPF 30** means that sunscreen filters out 97 percent of the sun's UVB rays, and **SPF 50** means the sunscreen protects against 98 percent of the sun's UVB rays.

Sunscreens with an SPF lower than 15 must now include a warning on the label stating that the product has been shown only to help prevent sunburn, not skin cancer or early aging of the skin.

The difference between SPF 30 and SPF 50 is only 1 percent. That's why, the higher SPF number doesn't mean that it's a lot better. And, no sunscreen protects you 100 percent. So, I recommend that you don't spend extra money on sunscreen that has an SPF of greater than 50.

Water-resistant sunscreen: There's actually no such thing as waterproof sunscreen because sweat and water wash any sunscreen off our skin. In fact, the FDA no longer allows manufacturers to claim that a sunscreen is waterproof. However, you can look for sunscreens that have a water-resistant label. This label describes how long (either 40 or 80 minutes) the sunscreen will stay on wet skin. The "40 minutes" label designates water-resistant sunscreen. Those labeled "very water resistant" are those that can stay on wet skin for 80 minutes. Those sunscreens labeled "sport" are usually water-resistant.

Even if your skin remains dry while you are using a water-resistant sunscreen, you'll need to reapply the sunscreen every 2 hours if you want to stay in the sun continuously for more than that. This is especially important when it comes to vacation or leisure time. If you spend time at the swimming pool or beach, swimming, toweling and bathing can wash the sunscreen off more quickly than you might realize. Nevertheless, a water-resistant sunscreen will help you protect yourself from the sun damage.

Chemical versus physical sunscreen: Chemical sunscreen protects your skin differently from physical sunscreen. Chemical sunscreen protects you by absorbing the sun's rays while physical sunscreen protects you by deflecting the sun's rays. The two ingredients of physical sunscreens are titanium dioxide and zinc oxide. They are inert, so they offer a much lower possibility of causing allergic reactions in those who use them. This is useful for people with sensitive skin or those who suffer from rosacea or other conditions exacerbated by heat. These ingredients in your sunscreen stop the sun's UV rays from passing through and entering the skin.

The physical sunscreen products do stop both UVA and UVB rays, so they offer a broad spectrum of sun protection for you. They offer immediate protection, so, as soon as you apply them, you can go out into the sun safely. This is one of the reasons they are found in many standard sunscreen products. They last longer on the shelf because the ingredients are inert, so you can keep on storing them and using them for a longer period of time.

One major disadvantage to a zinc oxide sunscreen that probably prevents many people from using it: It gives the skin a pasty white appearance and is very visible.

The list of ingredients in chemical sunscreen ingredients is a lot longer. These ingredients attract the rays of the sun and convert them into heat and release that heat from the skin.

Chemical sunscreen tends to be thinner than physical sunscreens, so they spread more easily on the skin. This means they are easier to apply, and you need a lesser amount of them. Chemical sunscreen is also less likely to leave gaps where the skin is exposed and unprotected.

The disadvantage of using chemical sunscreen is that, unlike physical sunscreen, it requires about 20 minutes after application before it begins to work, and application can cause greater chances of irritation. This is especially important to note for those with sensitive skin.

Physical Sunscreen
i.e. zinc oxide and titanium dioxide

Chemical Sunscreen
i.e. avobenzone

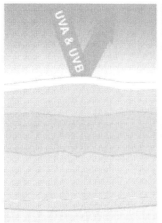
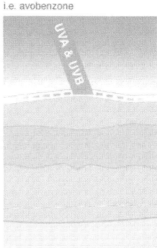

Image from: http://www.acne.org/spf-sunscreen.html

Included in this section of my book is a table from skincancer.org, showing us different types of sunscreen ingredients that are approved by the FDA. The table also differentiates between chemical or physical sunscreen and indicates which types of UV rays they protect against.

So, now when you choose a sunscreen, make sure you choose the ingredients that can provide you with both UVA and UVB protection. Some sunscreens on the market will also contain both chemical and physical sunscreen.

The bottom line: You want to have both UVA and UVB protection. Don't be fooled by the brand or the packaging. Just look at the ingredient list.

FDA-Approved Sunscreens	
Active Ingredient/UV Filter Name	**Range Covered** UVA1: 340-400 nm UVA2: 320-340 nm UVB: 290-320 nm
Chemical Absorbers:	
Aminobenzoic acid (PABA)	UVB
Avobenzone	UVA1
Cinoxate	UVB
Dioxybenzone	UVB, UVA2
Ecamsule (Mexoryl SX)	UVA2
Ensulizole (Phenylbenzimiazole Sulfonic Acid)	UVB
Homosalate	UVB
Meradimate (Menthyl Anthranilate)	UVA2
Octocrylene	UVB
Octinoxate (Octyl Methoxycinnamate)	UVB
Octisalate (Octyl Salicylate)	UVB
Oxybenzone	UVB, UVA2
Padimate O	UVB
Sulisobenzone	UVB, UVA2
Trolamine Salicylate	UVB
Physical Filters:	
Titanium Dioxide	UVB, UVA2
Zinc Oxide	UVB,UVA2, UVA1

Table from: http://www.skincancer.org/prevention/uva-and-uvb

For children, the American Academy of Dermatology (AAD) recommends using physical sunscreen on toddlers and babies older than 6 months. These are titanium dioxide and zinc oxide; they are less likely to irritate a baby's sensitive skin. For children younger than 6 months old, it is recommended that they avoid the sun and using sunscreen altogether. Keep children in the shade and dress them in clothing that will protect their skin from the sun (that is, long-sleeved shirts, pants, and wide-brimmed hats).

Those with sensitive skin should choose the "sensitive" labeled sunscreen because these sunscreens will contain titanium dioxide or zinc oxide; they are less likely to irritate the skin. Chemical sunscreens tend to irritate more if you have sensitive skin.

Many products claim to be hypoallergenic or dermatologist-tested, but the only way to know for sure if a product will irritate your skin is to check its ingredients and try it. One common recommendation is to apply a small amount to the soft skin on the inside of your elbow every day for 3 days. If your skin does not turn red or become itchy, the product is probably okay for you to use.

Don't use sunscreen that contains insect repellant: While both sunscreen and insect repellant are important, how much of each is needed is different. With sunscreen, we need to use a lot and reapply it every 2 hours. Insect repellant, on the other hand, should be applied sparingly and less often than sunscreen. Therefore, it is best to buy these products separately.

Spray, powder, or cream form? Sunscreen is meant to be applied to our skin. I recommend that you don't spray the sunscreen onto your skin because you can inhale the chemicals it contains. The cells in our lungs are different from those on our skin, so how our lungs react to the chemicals will be different from how our skin does.

Therefore, it's best to apply sunscreen on our skin using our hand rather than by spraying it. However, if you have a spray can bottle of sunscreen, you can spray it on your hand first and then apply it on your skin. Same goes for those that contain powder sunscreen. The loose powder can be inhaled into our lungs. If you must use these powders, make sure to hold your breath while applying them to your skin.

A word about expiration dates: Check the expiration date on the sunscreen to be sure it's still effective. Most sunscreen products are good for at least 2 to 3 years, but you may need to shake the bottle to remix the sunscreen ingredients. Sunscreens that have been exposed to heat for long periods may be less effective.

How to use sunscreen properly

Always follow the label directions. Most recommend applying sunscreen generously. When putting it on, pay close attention to your face, ears, neck, arms, and any other areas not covered by clothing. If you're going to wear insect repellent or makeup, put the sunscreen on first.

As a rule, apply an SPF 30 or higher sunscreen 30 minutes before you go outside, so the product has time to soak into your skin and provide the maximum benefit. You should apply sunscreen every day, even if it is cloudy. Ideally, about 1 ounce of sunscreen (about a shot glass or palmful) should be used to cover the arms, legs, neck, and face of the average adult.

Sunscreen needs to be reapplied at least every 2 hours to maintain protection. Sunscreens can wash off when you sweat or swim and then wipe off with a towel, so they might need to be reapplied more often. Be sure to read the label. And don't forget your lips; lip balm with sunscreen is also available to purchase.

Reminder about what this book is all about

The best way to look after your skin from start to finish is to be informed about what you actually need and to make the best use of that wherever you can. The purpose of this book is to help you with your education when it comes to your skin. The book is also a good start in creating your skincare plan because it shows you the different ingredients that you need to look out for in your quest to have healthy skin that doesn't age long before the rest of your body.

Just as with choosing skin creams, you need to look at the ingredients listed on sunscreen bottles when you next make a selection and determine whether this product is going to provide you with the protection you need.

The answers don't lie in the promotion, the sales assistant's recommendation or a celebrity endorsement. **The answer lies in the list of ingredients and your new-found knowledge of what the different ingredients can do for you.**

Don't take shortcuts in the selection because the protection you provide for your skin pays off in the long term.

The skin that is looked after is the skin that will still look great when you get older. This is what you want for yourself. Start today by making these changes: **Stay out of the sun and use sunscreen when you do go out**. These are the two most important steps you can take on your road to great skin.

Moisturizers

The purpose of moisturizers is to hold water in the outermost layer of skin. They also act as a temporary barrier against environmental pollution. As I mention throughout the book, keeping our skin moisturized and hydrated and preventing pollution exposure are important methods of slowing the skin's aging process. Therefore, knowing which moisturizers to use for what purpose is very important. Unfortunately, the number of moisturizers available on the market today is quite staggering, so let me tell you a little about the three main types and how they can work for you.

The 3 types of moisturizers are emollients, humectants, and occlusives. **Emollients** help soothe and soften the skin and increase moisture levels in the skin, and they come in the form of ointment, cream, lotion, or gel. They act as a barrier, so they are often used to alleviate dryness, and for routine skincare. **Squalene** is one of the most common lipids produced by human skin cells and is a component of human sebum; therefore, it is a great natural emollient. Unfortunately, the production of squalene slows drastically after age 30, thus contributing to dry skin. It can be derived from both plant and animal sources and is often included as an ingredient in skincare creams.

Humectants are natural or synthetic chemicals that attract and retain water in the epidermis, the top layer of the skin. They attract water two ways: from the dermis or from the environment. **Glycerin** is the most effective humectant. **Urea**, if used at less than 10 percent, is a humectant, but if used at 20 to 30 percent, will cause shedding of the skin. Because humectants draw water from the dermis into the epidermis, their use will actually decrease overall skin hydration; water will evaporate from the upper layer of the skin. Therefore, humectants are often used with occlusives to prevent water loss. You should also drink plenty of water to maintain hydration for your body overall.

Occlusives are oils and waxes that form a physical block on the skin to prevent water loss. Of all the different occlusives, **petrolatum** provides the best protection and prevention of water loss, followed by **lanolin**, then **mineral oil**. Therefore, keep a jar of petrolatum jelly in your house in case you ever need to prevent water loss from your skin on those days that your skin feels dry.

Unfortunately, occlusives increase the risk of acne breakouts.

Now that you have a better idea of how the 3 types of moisturizers work, it's important to note that you might find the ingredients of all 3 types of moisturizers listed on the label of an individual skincare product. This table displays, at a glance, the properties of the 3 types of moisturizers.

Types of Moisturizers	Emollients	Humectants	Occlusives
How they work	Create skin barrier	Attract water to epidermis	Act as a physical block
Uses	Dry skin and routine care	Dry skin	Dry skin, eczema, prevention of contact irritation
Side effects	Rarely	Irritation (urea, lactic acid)	Messy to apply, increase acne risk
Ingredients	Cholesterol, squalene, fatty acids, fatty alcohols, pseudocera mides	Glycerin, propylene glycol, butylene glycol, panthenol sorbitol, urea <10%, alpha hydroxyl acids (i.e., glycolic or lactic acid), hyaluronic	Petrolatum, paraffin, caprylic/ca pric triglyceride, squalene, lanolin acid, stearic acid, cetyl alcohol, stearyl alcohol, lanolin,

		acid, sodium pyrrolidine carboxylic acid, aluminum lactate and sodium lactate, gelatin, honey	lecithin, propylene glycol, cholesterol, carnauba, candelilla, beeswax, mineral oil, silicones, stearyl stearate, lanolin, zinc oxide

It is useful to know the different forms moisturizers come in and how they can help you with your skin conditioning. Too much moisture in the skin can also be a bad thing, so make sure you use a moisturizer appropriate for your need.

The moisturizer that's best for you depends on many factors, including your skin type, your age and whether you have specific conditions, such as acne. People with oily skin are prone to acne and breakouts, so they need to choose a water-based product, such as a gel that's labeled "noncomedogenic", which means it won't clog pores. For people with normal or combination skin, which is neither too oily nor too dry, a lotion is fine. And people with dry skin need to choose a cream form because it has more occlusives (increased oil and wax content). This will prevent the loss of water.

Those with extremely dry skin need to use an ointment form of moisturizer because it will be petrolatum based. However, a petrolatum-based moisturizer will be very greasy and can clog pores and cause acne. As for sensitive skin, it is susceptible to skin irritations, redness, itching and/or rashes. Look for a moisturizer that contains soothing ingredients, such as chamomile or aloe, and doesn't contain potential allergens, such as fragrances or dyes. Also, avoid products containing acids, which can irritate sensitive skin.

For mature skin, you need to choose a cream form or ointment form because, as you age, your skin tends to become drier because your oil-producing glands become less active. Again, only use ointment if your skin is extremely dry.

The different forms moisturizers come in are shown in the table provided here:

Form	Description	Skin Type
Gel	High water content Lowest wax and oil content	Oily skin
Lotion	High water content	Normal/ combination skin
Cream	Higher oil and wax content Creates occlusive layer that replaces and retains water	Dry skin, mature skin

Ointment	Greasy Clog pores, cause acne No preservatives required	Extremely dry skin

How to use moisturizers to best effect

Moisturizers are best when used immediately after bathing. So, after a bath, pat or blot your skin until it's just barely dry, then apply moisturizer immediately within 10 minutes for better absorption into the skin. Also, don't forget to apply moisturizer to your hands and body as needed. Your hands get more exposure to irritants than do any other body parts, so make sure you apply moisturizer to your hands after a bath or after you wash your hands.

Now that you know different types of moisturizers, and which form is best for you, remember that, as we have discussed elsewhere in this book, buying the most expensive moisturizer is not the way to go. Understand which ingredients serve your purpose and which form of moisturizer best fits your needs. Keep in mind that your skin changes due to many factors, so choose the right moisturizer for your specific skincare needs.

Cleansers

We cannot talk about moisturizers without talking about cleansers. After a long day during which our skin is exposed to pollution, we need to use a good cleanser to wash away all of the pollutants on our skin.

In my research on this topic, I didn't find a lot. However, one tip I want to leave with you is that your skin is naturally slightly acidic, with a pH of about 5. Therefore, you want to choose a gentle, nonabrasive cleanser that's pH balanced. If you choose cleansers that are not close to pH 5, you can throw off the balance of your skin, causing it to be drier, oilier and/or more prone to acne.

If you don't know your cleanser's pH levels and want to verify them for yourself, purchase pH papers online and test out your own cleansers. While you're at it, test out all of your skincare products and see what pH they may have. It will be a fun and eye-opening experiment for you. Some websites also provide reported pH levels of different brands of cleansers.

I cannot verify the accuracy of the **information on pH levels** offered on these websites, but you can find them here:

- https://docs.google.com/spreadsheets/d/1VqO_uF8m4oKBzzk5ass37gHcjIk-_2Tv4W2KgJJmUQc/edit
- http://www.dianayvonne.com/content/pHcleansers.pdf

Some cleansers also contain ingredients that are emollients, humectants, or exfoliants (which I will talk about in Chapter 4). I think having other good ingredients in your cleanser is good, but don't spend too much money on them. Cleansers are meant to clean your face, not act as a nutrient supplement for your skin. Your skincare cream will do that for you.

Choose a pH balanced gentle cleanser that has the ingredients you need. You should use a cleanser at least once a day, especially after you get home from being outside because your skin is exposed to pollution and dirt outside. If your face is dirty often, wash or rinse it more often. However, do not scrub your face because that will dry it out and cause more damage to your skin. Instead, gently rub in the cleanser and rinse with warm water. Also avoid using a washcloth or sponge, which can be rough enough to irritate the skin.

After you use a cleanser, apply a moisturizer right away to lock in the moisture of your skin. It will be better if your moisturizer also contains antioxidants to replenish the loss of antioxidants your skin uses to combat the pollution attacking your skin.

This brings us to our next set of wonderful ingredients that should be in your skincare creams, antioxidants!

Antioxidants

In addition to sunscreen and moisturizers, other ingredients will have a positive effect on your skin. The next group we will be looking at is the antioxidants contained in some skincare products, which can help you look after your skin and prevent the signs of premature aging.

At the beginning of this chapter, we talked about getting antioxidants into our body with proper nutrition. However, we also need to apply antioxidants directly on our skin because local application has more impact in terms of preventing aging.

Specifically, we are looking at vitamins C and E and green tea to help us maintain a youthful skin, fight against the damage of reactive oxygen species, and prevent the formation of wrinkles. You have probably heard of many different antioxidants the media promotes for skincare use. However, I choose to focus on the two vitamins because they are naturally occurring antioxidants in our skin, they decrease as we age, and clinical data supports their use in skincare cream to prevent aging skin. Green tea also has clinical data supporting its use as an antioxidant with protective properties.

Vitamin C

Vitamin C is an important antioxidant and a vital nutrient for human diet. It is important for your skin, bones, and connective tissue. It promotes healing and helps the body absorb iron. There are many names and forms of vitamin C, as follows: Acide Ascorbique, Acide Cévitamique, Acide Iso-Ascorbique, Acide L-Ascorbique, Acido Ascorbico, Antiscorbutic Vitamin, Ascorbate, Ascorbate de Calcium, Ascorbate de Sodium, Ascorbyl Palmitate, Calcium Ascorbate, Cevitamic Acid, Iso-Ascorbic Acid, L-Ascorbic Acid, Magnesium Ascorbate, Palmitate d'Ascorbyl, Selenium Ascorbate, Sodium Ascorbate, Vitamina C, Vitamine Antiscorbutique, Vitamine C. When you see these ingredients on the side of the packaging for skincare product, you know they contain vitamin C. However, **ascorbic acid** is the most studied form of vitamin C, and it has the least number of side effects.

Clinical studies show that vitamin C can increase collagen production, protect against damage from UVA and UVB rays, correct pigmentation problems, and improve inflammatory skin conditions. Because vitamin C is an antioxidant, it helps neutralize all the bad free radicals that can damage your skin. That's why it is a great protective ingredient. It is a skin lightener, so if you have dark spots or sun damage, a skin cream with vitamin C will help you feel better about the way your skin looks overall.

Vitamin C is another ingredient that actually increases collagen production in the skin, so you get more of that component of the skin that provides strength and elasticity. Because of this, it actually reduces the appearance of wrinkles on your skin and halts the aging process. This is a huge positive when you are looking to have healthy skin for a long time.

Vitamin C as ascorbic acid has a natural anti-inflammatory effect on the skin, so the damage that may be happening from inflammation will be stopped, and you can get on with having great skin. This is one of the reasons that vitamin C is often added to sunscreens so that you experience its anti-inflammatory effects when you are out in the sun.

Studies show that products containing 5 to 10 percent of vitamin C do not cause irritation or redness. However, vitamin C can be unstable as an ingredient in a cream. With time, it will turn yellow or close to brown due to oxidation. If you use skin cream containing vitamin C, look for containers that seal out air so that your vitamin C doesn't get oxidized easily.

Creams containing vitamin C can feel sticky on your skin. For those who don't like that sticky feeling, it's best to apply vitamin C at night, so you don't have to feel that sticky feeling during the day.

What we've learned so far about vitamin C as an ingredient in skin cream
Vitamin C is an ingredient that will help you in many areas of your skincare regimen because it aids in the fight against

aging skin and the underlying causes of that aging without the need for injections or surgery.

Remember the effects that vitamin C can have as an ingredient in skin cream.

- **Lightens the skin**
- **Increases collagen production**
- **Reduces the appearance of wrinkles**
- **Anti-inflammatory**

Vitamin E

Vitamin E is an oil-soluble anti-oxidant that can help the skin in many ways. It can be found in different forms with many names: Acétate d'Alpha Tocophérol, Acétate d'Alpha Tocophéryl, Acétate de D-Alpha-Tocophéryl, Acétate de DL-Alpha-Tocophéryl, Acétate de Tocophérol, Acétate de Tocophéryl, Acétate de Vitamine E, All-Rac-Alpha-Tocophérol, All Rac-Alpha-Tocopherol, Alpha-Tocophérol, Alpha Tocopherol Acetate, Alpha Tocopheryl Acetate, Alpha Tocotriénol, Bêta-Tocotriénol, Bêta-Tocophérol, Concentré de Tocotriénol, D-Alpha Tocopherol, D-Alpha Tocophérol, D-Alpha Tocopheryl Acetate, D-Alpha-Tocopherol, D-Alpha-Tocophérol, D-Alpha-Tocophéryl, D-Alpha-Tocopheryl Acetate, D-Alpha Tocopheryl Acetate, D-Alpha-Tocophéryl, D-Alpha-Tocopheryl Acid Succinate, D-Alpha-Tocopheryl Succinate, D-Alpha Tocotrienol, D-Alpha Tocotriénol, DL-Alpha-Tocopherol, DL-Alpha-Tocopheryl, DL-Alpha-Tocopheryl Acetate, D-Tocopherol, D-Tocopheryl Acetate, DL-Tocopherol, D-Beta-Tocopherol, D-Bêta-Tocophérol, D-Delta-Tocopherol, D-Delta-Tocophérol, Delta-Tocotriénol, Delta-Tocophérol, D-

Gamma-Tocopherol, D-Gamma Tocotrienol, D-Gamma-Tocotriénol, D-Gamma-Tocophérol, DL-Alpha-Tocophérol, DL-Alpha-Tocophéryl, DL-Tocophérol, D-Tocophérol, Fat-Soluble Vitamin, Gamma-Tocotriénol, Gamma-Tocophérol, Mixed Tocopherols, Mixed Tocotrienols, Palm Tocotrienols, Rice Tocotrienols, RRR-Alpha-Tocopherol, RRR-Alpha-Tocophérol, Succinate Acide de D-Alpha-Tocophéryl, Succinate Acide de Tocophéryl, Succinate de D-Alpha-Tocophéryl, Succinate de Tocophéryl, Succinate de Vitamine E, Tocopherol, Tocopherol Acetate, Tocophérols Mixtes, Tocopheryl Acetate, Tocopheryl Acid Succinate, Tocopheryl Succinate, Tocotrienol,Tocotriénol, Tocotrienol Concentrate, Tocotriénols, Tocotrienols, Tocotriénols de Palme, Tocotriénols de Riz, Tocotriénols Mixtes, Vitamin E Acetate, Vitamin E Succinate, Vitamina E, Vitamine E, Vitamine Liposoluble, Vitamine Soluble dans les Graisses.

When you look at the packaging of your skincare products, and you come across these names, you know the product contains a form of vitamin E. You will often find products containing vitamin E at a level from 0.5 to 5 percent.

Vitamin E has fewer beneficial properties for skincare than the other vitamins but is nonetheless an important part of your skincare regimen. It has healing properties that help the skin prevent and reverse damage caused by UV rays. It is especially useful for treating sunburn, UV-induced redness, skin photo-aging that presents itself in the form of wrinkles, and hyper-pigmentation of the skin. It is an oily or greasy substance so may not be ideal for those who have problems with oily skin, but it will help to deal with the effects the sun and its harmful rays have on the skin.

Vitamin E can prevent skin problems caused by UV exposure as follows:

- **Sunburns**
- **UV-induced redness**
- **Skin photo-aging (wrinkles)**

Green tea

Green tea contains polyphenols, which are great antioxidants. The many names of green tea are as follows: Benifuuki, Constituant Polyphénolique de Thé Vert, CPTV, EGCG, Epigallo Catechin Gallate, Épigallo-Catéchine Gallate, Epigallocatechin Gallate, Extrait de Thé Vert, Extrait de Camellia Sinensis, Extrait de Thé, Extrait de Thea Sinensis, Green Sencha Tea, Green Tea Extract, Green Tea Polyphenolic Fraction, GTP, GTPF, Japanese Sencha Green Tea, Japanese Tea, Kunecatechins, Poly E, Polyphenon E, PTV, Té Verde, Tea Extract, Tea Green, Tea, Thé, Thé de Camillia, Thé Japonais, Thé Vert de Yame, Thé Vert, Thé Vert Sensha, Yabukita, Yame Green Tea, Yame Tea.

If you see these names listed among the ingredients in your skincare products, then they contain green tea. The most common form of green tea used in skin creams is **ECG** with a range of 0.1 to 2 percent.

Green tea is thought to be beneficial for preventing skin damage and cancer from ultraviolet (UV) radiation due to the antioxidant effects of the polyphenols it contains. Polyphenolic extracts of green tea, specifically EGCG and epicatechin-3-gallate, when used on the skin, seem to protect against UVA and UVB sunburn. Green tea extracts also seem to prevent UV radiation-induced DNA damage.

The bottom line: Green tea is beneficial for **preventing skin damage and cancer from UV rays.**

Other antioxidants

As you now realize, the whole theme of prevention is focused on the prevention of damage from UV rays and the breakdown of collagen and elastin. Other ingredients can help with this type of prevention.

Ingredients that help to prevent damage from UV rays include: **glutathione peroxidase, superoxide dismutase and catalase, glutathione (GSH), uric acid, alpha-lipoic acid,** and **ubiquinol** (also known as **Coenzyme Q10**). These ingredients are found naturally in our skin and throughout our bodies and are all considered antioxidants. Their main function is to neutralize the free radicals produced by our own bodies or by UV rays, leading to prevention of collagen and elastin damage. If you see products containing these names, you know they will help prevent damage from free radicals.

Lip balm

Ever wonder why your lips look thinner as you get older? Although your lips look different from the rest of your skin, they're actually quite similar, and they also age and lose their plumpness due to a decrease in collagen and elastin. Therefore, just like the rest of your body, your lips also need protection.

Lips have the same three layers as the rest of your skin, but their outer layer of epidermis (called the **stratum corneum)** is thinner than in other areas of the skin. Also your lips don't have any sebaceous glands, the gland that secretes sebum to keep your skin moisturized. The only way your lips normally get moisture is from your saliva, so that's why they can easily become dry and chapped.

Armed with the information I already talked about in this book, what do you think you will need in your lip balm? You're right: your lip balm will need to contain occlusives and humectants to keep moisture in your lips. That's why you see that chapsticks are so thick. A lot of chapsticks are made from beeswax or petrolatum.

Also, you want to prevent degradation of collagen and elastin, so what do you think will help with this? Sunscreen! So, look for lips balms that have good sunscreen ingredients, moisturizing ingredients, and maybe even antioxidants. Now, your lips and the rest of your body are as protected as they can be.

CHAPTER 4: REVERSING THE SIGNS OF AGING SKIN

Now that we have discussed ways to prevent aging skin, we will discuss what we should do if we already see signs that our skin is aging. In this chapter we are going to take a look at the different ways you can stop and possibly reverse the signs of aging and age gracefully instead.

As with this entire book, the idea is to help you gain confidence in the knowledge you build, so you know what to look for and what you need to do to deal with the different changes in your skin. You already know that you will start seeing changes in your skin through intrinsic and extrinsic aging as you get older. Therefore, in this chapter, we will be focusing on the older population.

Lifestyle changes

The first step in treating aging skin is to prevent your skin from getting worse. Therefore, you need to make changes in your lifestyle, which I have already mentioned in Chapter 3 of this book. Those lifestyle changes are:

- Avoiding extreme temperatures
- Avoiding UV radiation
- Avoiding pollution
- Quitting cigarette smoking and avoiding secondhand smoke
- Adopting good nutrition habits by including antioxidant-rich, anti-inflammatory foods in your diet
- Getting adequate sleep

- Increasing water intake
- Decreasing alcohol intake
- Decreasing stress (and, thus, decreasing cortisol levels in your body)

The recommendation to avoid extreme temperatures, UV radiation, pollution, smoking and to decrease alcohol intake and stress levels are the same whether you're 20 years old or 60. However, sleeping is more difficult as you age. So, in this case, try for quality sleep instead of quantity. Make sure you get uninterrupted sleep, and the recommendation is to get both rapid eye movement (REM) and non-REM sleep to feel rested.

Increasing water intake can be a challenge for older people because many of them have conditions that require medication that causes them to lose water. People who have heart failure or conditions that require water restriction should consult with their health care professionals to determine how much liquid they can take in. The general rule does not apply to them.

As people age, they need fewer total calories, but more nutrients, especially protein, B-Vitamins and calcium. Therefore, one should focus on quality and not quantity when you select food. All your food choices, for every food group, need to be power-packed with more nutrients per calorie. Choose foods from all the MyPlate food groups.

You can find **information on the MyPlate food groups** on this website: http://www.choosemyplate.gov/.

Desired Ingredients	Examples of foods with a high amount of a desired ingredient
Protein	Eggs, milk, yogurt, fish and seafood, soy, pistachio nuts, chicken, and beans.
B-Vitamins • B1 (thiamine) • B2 (riboflavin) • B3 (niacin) • B5 (pantothenic acid) • B6 (pyridoxine) • B7 (biotin) • B9 (folic acid) • B12 (cyanocobalamine)	Fish, poultry, meat, eggs, and dairy products. Leafy green vegetables, beans, and peas also have B-vitamins.
Calcium	Dairy products, such as milk, cheese, and yogurt. Leafy, green vegetables. Fish with soft bones that you eat, such as canned sardines and salmon. Calcium-enriched foods, such as breakfast cereals, fruit juices, soy and rice drinks, and tofu.

You also need to eat food packed with proteins to maintain your muscle mass, fight infection and recover from an accident or surgery.

Here are **some tips from the Academy of Nutrition and Dietetics on how to increase your protein** intake:

- **"Enjoy More Beans.** Add canned beans to salads, soups, rice dishes and casseroles.
- **Make Your Crackers Count.** Spread peanut butter on your crackers and eat them alongside soup, chili or salad.
- **Pump Up Your Eggs.** Mix grated, low-fat cheese or extra whites into scrambled eggs.
- **Cook with Milk.** Use fat-free or low-fat milk rather than water to make soup or oatmeal.
- **Use Dry Milk Powder.** Mix a spoonful of dry milk into fluid milk, cream soups and mashed potatoes."

Not only do you need to increase your protein intake as you age to maintain your weight and your muscle mass, you need to do exercises.

According to the National Institute on Aging:

"There are four main types [of exercises] and each type is different. Doing them all will help you benefit from the best effects of all of them:

- Endurance, or aerobic, activities increase your breathing and heart rate. Brisk walking or jogging, dancing, swimming, and biking are examples.

- Strength exercises make your muscles stronger. Lifting weights or using a resistance band can build strength.
- Balance exercises help prevent falls.
- Flexibility exercises stretch your muscles and can help your body stay limber."

Remember how, in Chapter 2, I mentioned that decreased muscle mass is one thing that causes wrinkles? If you don't have the muscle mass to hold up your skin, your skin can sag and start to have wrinkles. The best way to gain muscle mass is to exercise and increase protein in your diet!

There are a lot of articles written about building muscle in your body. Given this book's focus on helping your skin age gracefully, I want to give you some tips to build muscle in your face.

Did you know there are more than 50 muscles in your face? Skinny and older people don't have a lot of muscle mass in their face. This can cause them to look gaunt and older than they are.

Doing facial exercises will help tone up your face and help you look younger.

According to "How to Exercise Facial Muscles" from **WikiHow** and "Facial Exercises to Look Younger and Get a Muscular Jawline" from *Men's Fitness*, the following exercises help build muscle mass in your face.

Exercising Your Forehead and Eyes (from WikiHow: "How to Exercise Facial Muscles")

"1. **Pull on your forehead with your index finger.** Using just your fingers, you can apply pressure to your forehead so that shifting your eyebrows can strengthen that part of your face. This can help smooth lines on your forehead.

- o Put your index fingers just above each of your eyes.
- o Pull down on your eyes while trying to raise your eyebrows.
- o Repeat 10 times to help firm your forehead.

2. **Push your forehead with your hands.** This simple exercise uses your palms to create resistance while flexing your eyebrows. Doing this workout will help create smooth lines on your forehead.

- o Place each of your palms on the sides of your forehead, the bottom of each palm resting on your eyebrows. Your palms should be holding the skin firmly in place.
- o Raise your eyebrow muscles, like you are surprised, then lower them, like you are angry.
- o Raise and lower 10 times, then raise and hold for 30 seconds. Lower and hold for 30 seconds, then repeat the up and down against 10 more times.

3. **Do brow lifts.** Using your fingers and your eyebrows, you can exercise the muscles in your forehead. Just a little bit of pressure can create enough resistance for a good exercise.

- o Using two fingers in a peace sign, place your fingernails over each eyebrow.

- o Gently push that skin down with your fingers, then push your brows up and down.
- o Repeat the up and down motion with your brows 10 times.
- o Do 3 sets of 10, take a short rest, then do another 3 sets of 10.

4. Stretch your eyelids. Your eyelids are easy muscles to work, and don't need much resistance. Using your fingers can help you stretch them out, removing wrinkles and giving you stronger eyelids.

- o Sit down and close your eyes.
- o With your lids relaxed, use your index fingers to lift up your eyebrows. While lifting, keep your eyes closed to stretch your eyelids as far as possible.
- o Hold this position for 10 seconds, then relax and repeat 10 times.

5. Do an eye squeeze. Work your eyelids further by squeezing your eyes shut with a little stretching resistance from your mouth. Because it uses so many different muscles, this exercise can help to stretch out your entire face, not just your eyes.

- o Pull your lips downward so that your facial muscles tighten, then pull your lips to one side.
- o Squeeze one eye shut for one second, then repeat 10 times, holding your lips to the side. Then do the other eye.
- o Do 3 sets of 10 for each eye, take a short rest, then do another 3 sets of 10.

6. **Stretch your face while holding your eyes**. This will help to build the muscles around your eyelids to give you more awake-looking eyes. Use your fingers to provide some resistance to the basic action of opening and closing your eyes.

- o Make a C around your eyes using your thumbs and index finger. Make sure your index finger is over your eyebrow and thumb against your cheek.
- o Shut your eyes, and slowly squeeze your eyelids close together. Relax the tension without opening your eyes
- o Repeat squeezing and relaxing your eyelids 25 times.

Exercising Your Mouth

"1. **Exercise by smiling**. One of the simplest ways to firm up your smile is to practice doing it. In this exercise, you'll slowly move your mouth into the position of a full smile, holding different positions. This will give you better control of your face and smiling capabilities.

- o Slowly begin to smile by stretching the corner of your mouth laterally, lips still together.
- o After that, turn your mouth upward to expose your upper teeth.
- o Smile as widely as you can, displaying your teeth.
- o Once you have reached that point, slowly relax your mouth, bringing the smile back to the starting point.

o Stop at several stages on this expansion of your smile, and hold that position for 10 seconds.

2. **Apply pressure to your smile**. Similar to the last exercise, this one uses different stages of your smile to work the muscles in your face. Here, your fingers will provide extra resistance to further work the muscles around your mouth.

o Make a full smile, and use your fingers to hold it in place by putting pressure on each corner.
o Close your lips halfway, then fully, using your fingers to resist the movement.
o Hold each position for 10 seconds.

3. **Do a face lift exercise**. This exercise works the muscles around your upper lip to help prevent sagging and keep a strong lip contour. Doing it properly will help you have a stronger smile that shows more of your upper teeth.

o Open your mouth slightly and flare your nostrils. Wrinkle up your nose as far as possible, then slowly draw your upper lip as high as you can, and hold for 10 seconds.
o Leave your mouth slightly open, and place one finger under the eye on the cheekbone. Curl your upper lip slowly upward, keeping finger pressure on your face. Hold for 10 seconds, then slowly return to the original position.

4. **Do a lip exercise**. This is a simple exercise that will help increase the blood flow to your lips. This will give the fleshier parts a healthier, livelier, and more natural color.

- o Open your mouth slightly, making sure your upper and lower lips are relaxed.
- o Bring your lower lip forward until it makes contact with your upper lip.
- o Bring your upper and lower lips inward to your mouth. Exert pressure, then relax.

5. **Do a mandibular strengthening exercise**. This exercise works your mandible, the lower jaw, an important part of smiling, talking, and chewing, as well as anything else your mouth does. An exercise like this will help to prevent a double chin and prevent aging grooves on the lower part of your face.

- o Keep your mouth, especially your teeth and lips, slightly closed.
- o Separate your teeth as much as you can without opening your lips.
- o Bring your mandible forward slowly. Go as far as you can, stretching your lower lip upward, and hold for 5 seconds.
- o Slowly return your jaw, lips, and then teeth, back to their original position.

6. **Do the OO-EE mouth**. Moving your mouth to some basic sounds can help you target the lips, as well as the muscles between your upper lip and nose. This is a simple exercise that only requires some exaggerated facial movement while making sounds.

- o Open your mouth, then purse your lips together so that your teeth are separated and not showing.
- o Say "OO," using an exaggerated movement to purse your lips together.
- o Change sounds to "EE," again using an exaggerated motion to stretch your lips into the proper shape. You can also replace "EE" with "AH" for a slightly different workout.
- o Do 10 reps between "OO" and "EE," then repeat for 3 sets.

7. **Suck on your finger**. Use the natural pressure from a sucking motion to firm up your lips. By removing it at the same time, you'll be able to provide additional resistance to work against.

- o Put your finger in your mouth, and suck on it as hard as possible.
- o While doing that, slowly remove it from your mouth.
- o Repeat 10 times.

8. **Press on your cheeks while smiling**. This will help strengthen your cheek muscles. Make sure to keep your head back when you do this exercise.

- o Press down on your cheeks with your three middle fingers.
- o While pushing, smile as hard as you can to push your fingers back.

9. **Pull your cheeks up**. This exercise can help smooth laugh lines and the fine lines around your under-eye. Your hands will be doing the work here,

stretching the muscles on your face and skin.

- o Place your palms firmly against your cheeks.
- o Pull the corners of your lips up toward your temples until you expose your upper teeth and gums.
- o Hold the position for 30 seconds, release, then repeat 3 times.

10. **Squeeze your lips**. This exercise will help to condition your lip muscles. Once again, your hands will do the work by squeezing your face around your mouth and nose.

- o Place your palms on your face, with the outer edge on your laugh lines and the bottom edges on the top of the jaw line. Use your whole palm to put pressure on your face.
- o Use your lip muscles (not your hands) to push your lips together and hold for 20 seconds. Then, push your palms up toward your nose and hold for 10 seconds.
- o Repeat the exercise 3 times."

Exercising Your Chin and Cheeks (from the *Men's Fitness* article "Facial Exercises to Look Younger and Get a Muscular Jawline")

1. "**Tongue Press**. This will target sagging underneath the chin.

- • Place your tongue on the roof of your mouth, right behind your teeth.
- • Then add tension by tightly pressing your tongue to completely close the roof of your mouth, and begin making the noises

"mh, mh, mh, mh." "It's very important to make the humming/vibrating sound when performing these exercises because they assist the muscles," says Georgesku.

- Do 3 sets of 10, rest, then another 3 sets of 10.

2. **Sagging Chin**. This will target underneath the chin and jawline area. Cleaves says if you execute these exercises for 15 minutes, no more than 3 to 5 times a week (in addition to using the right skincare products and getting plenty of rest) you'll see improvement in two weeks.

   - Place your elbow on a table with your fist under your chin.
   - Then try to open your mouth while exerting force with your wrist to create resistance.
   - Hold then release.
   - Do 3 sets of 10.

3. **Double Chin Slide**. This works underneath the chin.

   - Place the palm of your hand under your chin, and with your mouth closed, stretch your lower jaw down as far as you can.
   - Then, exert pressure with your palm as you slide your hand along the double chin area, the jawline, and the side of the face ending at your temples.
   - Do this 10 times (5 right and 5 left).

4. **Cheek Firmer**. This will work your cheek and jawline area.

- Place the length of your index finger below the eye along the upper cheekbones.
- Then open your mouth as wide as comfortable, curl your lips over your bottom teeth, and smile with the corners of your mouth to create flex, then release.
- Do this 40 times."

Ingredients in products used to treat aging skin

Now that you know what lifestyle changes you need to make, let's discuss what products (and their ingredients) you need to help reverse the signs of aging skin.

In terms of products, you will still need the ones mentioned in Chapter 3 of this book, so let's refresh our memories as to what those are: sunscreen, moisturizer, cleanser, and lip balm. In that chapter, we also pointed out that you'll want antioxidants in your cream that have protective properties: vitamin E, green tea, and especially vitamin C because, not only is it an antioxidant, it also promotes collagen production.

For the most part, antioxidants can only prevent, not reverse, the signs of aging. Wrinkles are formed when collagen breaks down, and skin dries out, thins and turns rough. Therefore, we need to look for ingredients that can stimulate collagen production so that the dermis will go back to its full thickness.

The dermis is the thickest layer of the skin with 90 percent made up of collagen. We also need ingredients that help to get rid of the dead skin layer that causes roughness, and we need to look for ingredients that increase our skin's hydration. I will concentrate on vitamin A, peptides, vitamin B3, hyaluronic acid, exfoliants, and skin-lightening agents. Clinical studies show the effectiveness of these ingredients in fighting aging skin.

Vitamin A

Vitamin A is a fat-soluble vitamin essential to our health. It helps us see in the dark, promotes normal growth and health of body cells, and keeps skin healthy. There are many chemical names for vitamin A that you may see: 3-Dehydroretinol, 3-Déhydrorétinol, Acétate de Rétinol, Antixerophthalmic Vitamin, Axerophtholum, Dehydroretinol, Déhydrorétinol, Fat-Soluble Vitamin, Oleovitamin A, Palmitate de Rétinol, Retinoids, Rétinoïdes, Retinol, Rétinol, Retinol Acetate, Retinol Palmitate, Retinyl Acetate, Rétinyl Acétate, Retinyl Palmitate, Rétinyl Palmitate, Vitamin A Acetate, Vitamin A Palmitate, Vitamin A1, Vitamin A2, Vitamina A, Vitamine A, Vitamine A1, Vitamine A2, Vitamine Liposoluble, Vitaminum A. If you see these names listed on the bottle's label, you know the cream contains vitamin A.

Vitamin A comes in different forms: retinol, retinal (also called retinaldehyde), retinoic acid, and retinyl esters. These different forms of vitamin A (synthetic or natural) are often collectively referred to as "retinoids". Vitamin A, also called retinol, cannot be synthesized by humans, so the only way to get vitamin A is through diet. The main dietary forms of pro-vitamin A include beta-carotene and retinyl esters. Metabolites of vitamin A include retinaldehyde and retinoic acid. The main transport form of vitamin A in the body is retinol, while retinoic acid is the biologically active form of vitamin A.

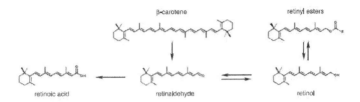

Retinol, retinaldehyde, and retinyl esters are considered precursors to the biologically active form, retinoic acid. Therefore, all the precursors are considered natural retinoic acid precursor and can be used in cosmetics while retinoic acid and all its synthetic derivatives are considered drugs and cannot be used in cosmetics.

Another name for retinoic acid is tretinoin, and some of its synthetic derivatives are isotretinoin (brand name is Acutane), adapalene, tazarotene. We will concentrate in this book on the natural retinoic acid precursors (retinyl esters, retinol, and retinaldehyde). You will find retinyl esters such as retinyl acetate, retinyl palmitate, and retinyl propionate in skincare cream.

There has been much research about retinoids, and retinoids help your skin in many ways because they can easily penetrate the epidermis. Retinoids have a protective role in that they absorb and filter UV radiation. They also help stimulate new skin generation in the epidermis.

Use of topical retinoids has been demonstrated to decrease discoloration due to age or sun damage. The application of a topical retinoid facilitates improved penetration of other topical bleaching agents, including hydroquinone. (I will talk about hydroquinone later in this chapter.) A decrease in fine and coarse wrinkling has been observed in topical retinoid users. It has been shown that topical retinoids improve the production of collagen and elastin, leading to reversal of wrinkles and skin laxity.

Retinoids also have anti-inflammatory effects, which is very beneficial for acne treatment, as well as for decreasing inflammation in photo-damaged skin. Improvement in skin texture is another benefit of retinoids. It increases hydration of the epidermis and dermis, as well as sebum secretion, which may alleviate dry skin and promote the skin's barrier function when paired with vitamin C in retinol peels. Retinoids also improve the physical connection between the epidermis and dermis, decreasing the skin's fragility caused by intrinsic aging or photo-damage.

The most common side effects of topical retinoids include redness, dryness, and itching. However, retinol and retinyl esters are not as irritating, but they are also not as effective as retinaldehyde. As you can see from the image of retinol included in this section of the book, retinaldehyde is just one step away from the active form, retinoic acid. Therefore, in terms of the best ingredient for skincare cream, retinaldehyde would be the best to have in your skincare cream, with 0.05 to 0.1 percent being the levels most tolerated with the least amount of irritation. However, you will find that most products have retinol or retinyl esters.

Another good way to get retinaldehyde is by consuming beta-carotene-rich food. So don't forget to eat food that's high in vitamin A or beta-carotene!

If your retinoid cream is causing irritation and redness, you can use aloe gel to help counter this effect because aloe gel is anti-inflammatory and helps with the itchiness caused by retinoids.

You will hear that it's not good to use retinoids when you are pregnant. To determine if something is safe to use for pregnancy, we have a pregnancy category system. Pregnancy categories are split into 4 different types: Category A is "generally acceptable", B is "may be acceptable", C is "use with caution if benefits outweigh risks", D is "use in life-threatening emergencies when no safe drug is available", and X is "do not use during pregnancy".

The confusing part of these categorizations is that vitamin A (retinol) and beta-carotene are naturally occurring and have been shown to be safe to consume in food. In fact, as an ingredient in our food, vitamin A is vital to our diet, so it is given pregnancy category A if taken as part of a woman's required daily consumption.

However, retinoic acid (the biological form of vitamin A) is given pregnancy category C, and the synthetic derivative of retinoic acid (isotretinoin) is given pregnancy category X. Synthetic derivatives of retinoic acid must definitely be avoided in pregnancy. Because retinoic acid is category C, and all the precursors lead to retinoic acid, it is better to avoid it if you are pregnant or planning to get pregnant.

What we've learned so far about retinoids

Retinoids perform some really key functions with respect to your skin. When I compiled a list of things that cause wrinkles, I found that many of them are countered by retinoids. They are a vital component of any good skin cream and will help you as you put together the list of ingredients you want and need from a skincare product. Make sure you look for them when you are choosing your next skin cream.

Retinoids help because of all of the important functions listed here:

- Protect skin from UV radiation
- Reduce fine lines and the appearance of wrinkles
- Reduce the breakdown of collagen
- Increase collagen production
- Reduce hper-pigmentation
- Increase skin hydration

Peptides

You can use this set of ingredients to help reverse the signs of aging. Throughout this book, you keep hearing about the importance of collagen and what an important role it plays in preventing wrinkles.

Collagen is like the cushion layer of a mattress. When the mattress is new, the cushion layer is bouncy and allows the fabric outside of it to remain smooth and taut. This is just like the relationship between collagen and skin.

The question is: Can you just add collagen into your skincare cream? Unfortunately, the collagen molecule is too large to slip through the epidermis to get to the dermis layer where it resides. There will be companies that claim that their cream contains collagen. However, it would be a waste of your money to buy because the collagen in the cream will not be able to get where it's needed. You can, however, get collagen directly by injecting it into the dermis layer, and I will discuss this approach later in this chapter.

In terms of using cream, the most effective way to increase skin collagen is to coax the body to produce more collagen on its own. Collagen is a protein that's made up of many amino acids. In turn, amino acids are considered the building blocks of proteins, and so proteins are your dietary source from which to obtain amino acids.

Without good nutrition that includes the appropriate amount of proteins, you will not get the building blocks required for your body to make and maintain collagen in your skin. When collagen breaks down, the long chains of amino acids turn into short chains of amino acids. These short chains of amino acids are called peptides. Peptides signal your body that there's a breakdown in collagen, and your body needs to make more.

Therefore, using synthetic peptides in your skincare cream is like tricking your body into thinking that there's not enough collagen in your skin and telling it to produce more. There are many peptides available. The common one most studied is palmitoyl pentapeptide-3 (also known as Matrixyl). It has been shown to stimulate new collagen production in the dermis layer of the skin. Another one commonly used in cosmetics is palmitoyl oligopeptide.

Another peptide is acetyl hexapeptide-3 (also known as Argireline®). Unlike the palmitoyl pentapeptide, acetyl hexapeptide acts similarly to botox, in that it inhibits neurotransmitters from being released from the nerves to the skin muscle. This prevents the contraction of face muscles, leading to your muscles relaxing and helping to reduce wrinkles. There are also other types of peptides that inhibit neurotransmitters and cause similar effects to those of Argireline®.

Please keep in mind that there are 20 types of essential amino acids that are the building blocks of our body's proteins. The cosmeceutical industry will use a combination of these amino acids to try to stimulate our skin or cause some kind of reaction in our skin. The name "peptide" can be misleading because the term just means a combination of amino acids.

However, only certain combinations will cause the effect you want. For example, the palmitoyl pentapeptide is the combination of palmitic acid with a 5-amino acid chain called lysine-threonine-threonine-lysine-serine. Palmitoyl oligopeptide contains palmitic acid with a 6-amino acid chain called valine-glycine-valine-alanine-proline-glycine.

Remember that I mentioned earlier in this book that the cosmetic industry is not well regulated? This lack of regulation can lead to mislabeling and cause consumers to be confused. Manufacturers don't have to tell you what type of amino acid is in their cream. All the labeling has to say is that it is a peptide. Look for products that contain the most researched (with real clinical studies) peptides. As we have seen, different combinations of different amino acids will cause different effects to your skin.

There are also new developments in the use of proteins, including plant-based proteins and growth factors in skincare cream. Plant-based proteins, such as soy or rice peptides, are used to correct skin pigmentation. Preliminary studies show that growth factors, such as transforming growth factors and fibroblast growth factors, can help reverse wrinkling.

Even though peptides have not been thoroughly studied yet, nor has their use in the skincare market been long, the future use of peptides or proteins will be interesting to follow.

Vitamin B3

Vitamin B3 is one of 8 B-Vitamins and comes in 2 forms: niacin (also known as nicotinic acid) and niacinamide (also known as nicotinamide). Chemical names you may see in a skincare cream are these: 3-Pyridine Carboxamide, 3-Pyridinecarboxylic Acid, Acide Nicotinique, Acide Pyridine-Carboxylique-3, Amide de l'Acide Nicotinique, Anti-Blacktongue Factor, Antipellagra Factor, B Complex Vitamin, Complexe de Vitamines B, Facteur Anti-Pellagre, Niacin-Niacinamide, Niacin/Niacinamide, Niacina y Niacinamida, Niacine, Niacine et Niacinamide, Nicamid, Nicosedine, Nicotinamide, Nicotinic Acid Amide, Nicotylamidum, Pellagra Preventing Factor, Vitamin PP, Vitamina B3, Vitamine B3, Vitamine PP.

In terms of what it does for the skin, vitamin B3 is another ingredient that can really help you get better skin. The most used form of vitamin B3 in skin cream is niacinamide. Like vitamin A, niacinamide can help the skin in many ways and help you look younger. Niacinamide has been shown to have anti-inflammatory and anti-microbial properties, and it reduces sebum production.

Because of its anti-inflammatory and anti-microbial effects, as well as its ability to help in reducing sebum production, niacinamide is listed as an ingredient in products that help with acne.

Niacinamide is also helpful for those with oily skin. In addition, it improves the natural skin barrier, which, in turn, helps improve your skin's texture. Niacinamide helps decrease histamine release and ultimately reduces itchiness. It also protects the skin from UV damage and has skin-lightening effects, which is of benefit to people who are starting to see age spots.

In conclusion, niacinamide carries out many functions that are really beneficial to the skin. It is another ingredient that will allow you to look after your skin and keep its appearance as young as possible for as long as possible.

The **ways that niacinamide helps you age gracefully** are as follows:

- Improves skin texture and increases its barrier properties
- Acts as an anti-inflammatory and anti-microbial
- Decreases oil production
- Has anti-histamine properties that reduce itching
- Reduces hyper-pigmentation/yellowing of skin
- Is photo-protective

Hyaluronic acid (HA)

Hyaluronic acid is a large sugar molecule in collagen-rich connective tissues and other tissues in our body. It has many functions, but in the skin, specifically, it attracts and binds water, therefore providing volume and fullness and maintaining skin's smoothness and moisture. As I mentioned earlier in this book, half of the hyaluronic acid in the human body is depleted by age 50 due to free radical damage. As we age, levels of hyaluronic acid in our skin also decreases. Therefore, we need to use cream that contains hyaluronic acid to supplement the loss of hyaluronic acid.

An interesting fact is that, even though we lose hyaluronic acid, this loss only pertains to the top layer of the skin, the epidermis. The hyaluronic acid level in our dermis layer doesn't change as we age. In fact, the amount of hyaluronic acid increases in our dermis layer when there is photo-damage.

The bottom line: As we age, we need to use moisturizers that contain hyaluronic acid to keep our skin hydrated and moisturized. Because hyaluronic acid is a natural chemical in our body, it is used as a dermal filler for our wrinkles as well, which I will talk about later in this chapter.

Exfoliants

Exfoliants have become very popular worldwide, especially in spas and for use at home, to remove the dead skin from the surface of your face. Without exfoliation, dead cells can build up on your skin; some of the cells can stay in the crevices of your wrinkles, making them look deeper than they actually are. So, when you lose these dead skin cells that are no longer needed, you allow new skin to generate and leave your face feeling smoother and younger as a result.

There are two basic ways to exfoliate: **physical scrub** and **chemical exfoliation**. A physical scrub is accomplished using a brush, bead, loofa, or other such scrubbing agent. These physical scrubs will physically scrape off the excess dead skin on your body. This method is great to use for your body, but I don't recommend a physical scrub for the face.

The skin on our face is very thin compared to the skin on the rest of our body. Using a physical scrub will increase the chances of damaging your facial skin if you scrub too hard. Also, with excess scrubbing, you will strip the skin of its natural oil, leaving your skin very dry.

The other way to exfoliate is to use ingredients that will help get rid of the skin's dead layer. The most used ingredients are hydroxy acids and salicylic acid. You will see that these ingredients can be found in facial masks, skincare cream, and even cleansers, and they all get rid of dead cells on your skin.

Hydroxy acids

Hydroxy acids come in four different types: alpha-hydroxy acids (AHAs), beta-hydroxy acids (BHAs), poly-hydroxy acids (PHAs), and bionic acids.

Many alpha-hydroxy acids (AHAs) are present in foods and fruits, and are often referred to as fruit acids. The common AHAs are glycolic and lactic acid. Glycolic acids are found in sugar cane, pineapple and cantaloupes. Lactic acids can be found in dairy products, such as yogurt, milk and fermented products. And again, in topical applications, these AHAs can often be found in peeling masks or cream.

The next type of hydroxy acids are the beta-hydroxy acids (BHAs). These are malic acid and citric acid, which can be found naturally in fruits. AHAs and BHAs both have anti-aging properties. They increase collagen production, hyaluronic acid, and skin thickness, and are helpful in lightening age spots. However, due to their acidic properties, AHAs can cause skin redness and irritation.

The next types of hydroxy acids that are less irritating than AHAs and BHAs are the poly-hydroxy acids (PHAs) and bionic acids (BAs). These are considered the next generation of hydroxy acids because they have similar anti-aging effects but cause less irritation. You will find the most common PHA ingredient in skincare cream is gluconolactone. The most common BA ingredient in skincare cream is lactobionic acid.

Hydroxy acids are the staple ingredients in skincare cream.

Hydroxy acid types	Example	Found in	Benefits/Uses
Alpha-hydroxy acids (AHAs)	Glycolic acid	sugar cane, pineapple, cantaloupes	Anti-aging (increased collagen, hyaluronic acid, and skin thickness), de-pigmentation, moisturizing, and as a peeling agent
	Lactic acid	dairy products, fermented products	
Beta-hydroxy acids (BHAs)	Malic acid	apple acid, watermelon	Antioxidant, anti-aging
	Citric acid	lemons, oranges, limes	
Poly-hydroxy acids (PHAs)	Gluconolactone	This is a metabolite our body makes	Anti-aging, strengthen the skin barrier, increase skin thickness, gentle moisturizing, antioxidant properties, less irritating than

			AHAs
Bionic acids (BAs)	Lactobionic acids	Lactose (found in the body and dairy products)	Attracts water to increase moisture, antioxidant properties, photo-damage prevention; more gentle, and less irritating than AHAs
	Maltobionic acids	Maltose (found in body and alcohol beverages)	
	Cellobionic acids	Cellobiose (resulting from the breakdown of cellulose, a natural fiber in food)	

Salicylic acid

Although salicylic acid is often thought to be a hydroxy acid because of its abilities as an exfoliating agent, its chemical structure is different from that of hydroxy acid, so it's not considered as such. When a cream containing salicylic acid is applied to the skin, the uppermost layer of skin swells, softens and peels, removing dead skin cells.

Salicylic acid is used to remove dark spots, acne and warts.

The amount of salicylic acid varies, depending on what it's used for.

Skin-lightening ingredients

Another sign of aging skin is age spots. Blemishes on our skin are due to intrinsic aging and also UV damage. Therefore, skin-lightening agents in skincare creams are very popular. I already mentioned retinoids (vitamin A), niacinamide (vitamin B3), vitamin C, salicylic acid, and also hydroxy acids.

Other ingredients that can lighten skin include **arbutin, kojic acid, alpha-lipoic acid** and **hydroquinone**. Hydroquinone is an ingredient available both over the counter (OTC) and by prescription in the U.S. The reason hydroquinone is regulated is because, even though it helps lighten the skin, exposure to sunlight or ultraviolet light will cause re-pigmentation of bleached areas in those who use hydroquinone and possibly make it worse. Chronic use leads to a discoloration of the nails, impaired wound healing, neuropathy, the so-called fish odor syndrome and exogenous ochronosis (a rare disease characterized by speckled and diffuse pigmentation symmetrically over the face, neck and photo-exposed areas).

Therefore, wearing sunscreen is required when you use hydroquinone. Currently, only up to 2 percent of hydroquinone is allowed in cosmetic cream, but there are products that have more than that 2 percent. You should use creams containing skin-lightening ingredients only at night, and you must wear sunscreen during the day.

Other ways to treat aging skin

Now that we have discussed different ingredients you can use in your skincare regimen, we will discuss other methods that go beyond nutrition and the ingredients contained in skincare products.

Hormone Replacement Therapy (HRT)

Hormone replacement therapy is useful when it comes to the hormones' effects on your skin. Loss of estrogen leads to loss of collagen and aging skin. Women who are going through menopause or who are post-menopausal will have a decrease in the levels of estrogen and progesterone.

Menopause is when a woman's menstrual periods permanently end. It happens any time from age 40 to age 59. It is a gradual process that can take a number of years and is a cause of intrinsic aging. Therefore, replacing lost hormones can be a way to combat intrinsic aging.

Hormone replacement therapy (HRT) is a treatment for menopause symptoms that involves taking synthetic hormones (which are made in a laboratory rather than by the body). These synthetic hormones can be bio-identical hormones or hormones derived from animals. Either way, HRT can be accomplished by taking estrogen alone or estrogen combined with another hormone, progestin.

Some women have found that HRT can relieve symptoms, such as hot flashes, vaginal dryness and some urinary problems. However, HRT is not for everyone. New information from recent studies suggests that, for most women, the risks of using HRT may outweigh the benefits. HRT is contraindicated in people with a personal or family history of breast/endometrial cancer, thromboembolism, recent undiagnosed genital bleeding or active severe liver disease. Talk to your doctor about the risks and benefits of

HRT before considering using it.

Note: There are skincare products on the market right now that do contain hormones in them, such as estradiol and progesterone. Make sure you read the ingredient list before you purchase!

Phytoestrogens may work in the body like a weak form of estrogen and can be used to relieve some symptoms of menopause. They are plant-based substances found in some cereals, vegetables, beans and other legumes, and herbs.

Many soy products, such as tofu, tempeh, soymilk and soy nuts, are good sources of phytoestrogens. Some studies indicate that soy supplements may reduce hot flashes in women after menopause. However, the results haven't been consistent.

There is not enough scientific evidence to recommend the use of herbs (creams or supplements) that contain phytoestrogens to treat symptoms of menopause. Herbs and supplements are not regulated in the way medicines are, and some herbs and supplements can be harmful when combined with certain medicines. If you're considering using any natural or herbal products for menopause, talk to your doctor first. It is best to get phytoestrogens through nutrition rather than in creams or supplements.

Microdermabrasion
In microdermabrasion, a special machine applies a slightly rough applicator tip (composed of tiny rough particles or a diamond tip) to the surface of the skin to remove the uppermost layer of skin. This results in a smoother skin

texture. The procedure is painless and non-invasive.

Multiple sessions of microdermabrasion may be required in some cases. Microdermabrasion is used to treat acne scars, sun-damaged skin, and wrinkles. Fortunately, the procedure is painless and typically no anesthetics are required. The only complications are skin irritation or possible infection. You must use moisturizer and sunscreen to protect your skin after microdermabrasion.

When you do microdermabrasion, make sure not to use chemical exfoliants or other physical scrubs at the same time because microdermabrasion acts like an exfoliant, removing the uppermost layer of skin. You don't want to cause too much exfoliation because it could lead to injury to your skin.

Dermal fillers (also known as wrinkle fillers, soft tissue fillers, or injectable implants)

Dermal fillers have gained in popularity as an alternative to going under the surgeon's knife with the potential pain and high cost that this can entail. As you would expect from the name, dermal fillers fill in the gaps in the skin where wrinkles occur. Although some skin creams claim to have wrinkle fillers, the preferred method of delivery is by injection of a substance under the skin.

Dermal fillers are also known as volumizers because they add volume and definition to the skin and can plump and lift jaw lines, cheeks, and temples; they can fill out thin lips and have even been known to be used to plump out the sagging skin on hands.

Most dermal fillers have a temporary effect because they contain materials that are absorbed by the body over time.

These temporary absorbable materials are collagen, hyaluronic acid, calcium hydroxylapatite, or Poly-L-lactic acid (PLLA). The FDA has approved only one product made from a material that remains in the body and not absorbed – polymethylmethacrylate beads (PMMA microspheres).

Some soft tissue fillers also contain lidocaine, which is intended to decrease pain or discomfort related to the injection. Dermal fillers made from absorbable (temporary) material are FDA-approved for the correction of moderate to severe facial wrinkles and skin folds, such as nasolabial folds. Nasolabial folds are the wrinkles on the sides of your mouth that extend towards the nose and are commonly referred to as "smile lines". The soft tissue filler made from non-absorbable (permanent) material is FDA approved ONLY for the correction of nasolabial folds. Other uses of dermal fillers are unapproved by the FDA and can cause unwanted complications.

As the name suggests, temporary dermal fillers don't last, so you have to go back and get another injection. Most side effects associated with soft tissue fillers happen shortly after injection and most go away in less than two weeks. Swelling and pain after hand treatment may last a month or more. In some cases side effects may appear weeks, months or years after injection.

There have been rare side effects reported to the FDA, and they are severe allergic reaction, migration/movement of filler material from the site of injection, leakage or rupture of the filler material at the injection site, and formation of permanent hard nodules on the face or hand, vision abnormalities including blindness, stroke, and damage to skin or lips.

Removing these fillers after they have been injected can be difficult. Therefore, make sure you are comfortable with the possible complications before you choose to have this procedure done.

Laser Skin Resurfacing

Laser skin resurfacing is a procedure that uses a laser to improve the appearance of skin or treat minor facial flaws by removing layers of skin. The two most common types of resurfacing lasers are **Carbon dioxide (CO2)** and **erbium**. Carbon dioxide is used to treat wrinkles, scars, warts and other conditions while erbium is used to remove superficial and moderately deep lines and wrinkles on the face, hands, neck and chest. Erbium causes fewer side effects than CO2 lasers.

Laser skin resurfacing will be carried out by a dermatologist or plastic surgeon and can take up to two hours for the whole face to be treated. It is quite an invasive way of treating the skin, so you will have to be bandaged immediately and those bandages will stay in place for the first 24 hours at least.

After the procedure, the skin can be prone to scarring or scabbing, so it will need to be cleaned 4 or 5 times a day and then you will also need to apply an ointment, such as petroleum jelly, to make sure that scabs do not form. Complications can include swelling, a burning sensation, itching, scarring, pigmentation issues, infection, and bumps due to obstruction of sweat glands. Healing takes 3 to 10 days, depending on the depth of the resurfacing and type of laser used. It is by far the most invasive of the methods we have looked at so far in this book.

Other treatment options

These other treatment options are invasive and severe courses of action. We started this book by looking at the ways to prevent your skin from aging prematurely. We have also looked at actions you can take, both in terms of limiting the effects of the extrinsic factors on your skin and in terms of the treatments that can help.

The bottom line: If you manage your skin, you don't need to take drastic action to improve the way it looks and the way you feel as you age. The ways that I have included here are for reference only.

In terms of this final set of options, I will only focus on Botox injections and cosmetic surgery. I recognize that there are other procedures available, such as light/laser therapy, dermabrasion, non-ablative laser rejuvenation, and the like.

Botox injections

Botox is a neurotoxin that, when injected, actually paralyzes the face muscles, thus softening the appearance of any wrinkles.

When Botox is injected into a muscle, it blocks the nerve signals that cause uncontrollable tightening and muscle movements. Botox is used to temporarily improve the look of both moderate to severe crow's feet lines and frown lines between the eyebrows in adults. The injections are regulated in most countries of the world, so you will need to visit someone who is trained, and more often than not, this will be a cosmetic (often referred to as "plastic") surgeon.

The medical professional should talk you through the procedure and make sure that you understand what you are about to go through and the potential risks associated with the procedure.

The potential side effects include the possibility of headaches, bruising and pain at the site of injection, and eye problems such as double vision, blurred vision, drooping and/or swelling of the eyelids.

Botox may also cause a life-threatening, serious side effect – the spread of toxin effects to other parts of the body. Botulinum toxin may affect areas away from the injection site and cause other serious symptoms, including loss of strength and all-over muscle weakness, double vision, blurred vision and drooping eyelids, hoarseness or change or loss of voice, trouble saying words clearly, loss of bladder control, trouble breathing, trouble swallowing. **Botox injections can result in loss of life**.

Cosmetic surgery

There are many types of cosmetic surgery for different parts of the body and all need to be carried out by a trained doctor who has passed all the relevant cosmetic surgery qualifications. Entering into surgery is never an easy decision, so you should seek medical advice, psychological counseling and the support of your friends and family if this is a course of action you are considering.

In terms of the types of cosmetic surgery to the face there are different options: a full face lift, neck lift, brow lift, or eyelid surgery. There are side effects and risks to any surgical procedure, and these are still true for cosmetic surgery.

A main risk is the potential for infection. Anesthesia risks (stroke being one of these) are also associated with the general anesthesia used during the procedure. Furthermore, where the incision is made, there is the strong potential that hair will not grow back. Of course this depends on where the scar is.

The scarring itself is also a potential side effect because, once the skin is cut, there is the very real possibility that the skin will scar permanently. Numbness or other changes in skin sensation are another risk.

There are psychological issues to explore when making any decision of this magnitude. The way you look helps define who you are to yourself, the people around you and society as a whole. The decision to have surgery should never be made lightly and should only be looked at as a last resort rather than a quick fix for your skin issue. Once you go through with the procedure, you cannot reverse it.

What we've learned so far in this book

The title of this book is *Age Gracefully: Make the Right Decisions for Your Skin*. I want you to learn the best ways to take care of your skin so that you can avoid these drastic measures and the potentially harmful side effects that they carry. This book is all about learning why and when to use what for your skin.

You learned why skin ages, how to prevent skin from aging, and what to use to prevent and treat aging skin. Therefore, you have learned how to make the right decisions for your skin and your loved ones. So the next chapter is all about putting a plan together to give you the tools you need so you can age gracefully and look your best.

CHAPTER 5: A STEPWISE APPROACH TO ANTI-AGING

As we have seen, there are many things to consider when it comes to taking care of your skin. Early in the book we learned about the factors that influence people's choice of skin cream. We looked at the marketing tactics, celebrity endorsements and free samples that dictate so many of our skincare product buying decisions.

As you read, many of us just keep trying new skin creams until we find one we think will work for us. The potential damage to our skin of trying out the wrong skin cream is an ever-present danger.

We have looked at the structure of the skin, its three layers and how they are formed. This has given us insight into how the layers perform and how they react to different stimuli. We have looked at the factors that will make our skin age. The intrinsic factors are always at play in our body and are part of the natural aging process. The extrinsic factors are outside factors that will age us prematurely.

Then we looked further into what causes wrinkles to form. Next, we looked at the protection that you should provide your skin. We considered ingredients that can help you and the treatment options you have. In this chapter we will pull all of this together to formulate a plan so that we all can age gracefully.

Before your skin begins to show signs of aging – 1st line intervention

Prevention is better than the cure with just about everything in life. With skincare it is absolutely essential to put in the work when you are young, so you can see the benefits as you get older. Parents with young children should teach your kids the principles of prevention of skin aging so that you will start them on a path to healthy and beautiful skin.

A lot of the principles of prevention are habits that should be instilled in all of us, especially in young children so that these habits are ingrained in them for life. It can be difficult when you are younger to start to think about what your skin will be like when you get older. By doing the right things early in life, you will have a positive impact on your skin's future.

Your skin needs to last you for a lifetime, so the measures you carry out now will pay off when you are older.

- **Habits important for prevention of aging skin:**

    - Avoiding extreme temperatures: not too hot or too cold

    - Avoiding exposure to UV radiation: outside and inside UV rays

    - Avoiding exposure to pollution

    - Quitting smoking and avoiding exposure to cigarette smoke

    - Maintaining good nutrition: plenty of antioxidant-rich and anti-inflammatory foods

- Getting adequate sleep

- Increasing water intake and maintaining proper hydration

- Decreasing alcohol intake

- Decreasing stress, thereby decreasing cortisol levels

- **Ingredients and products used to prevent skin aging:**

  - Sunscreen: physical and chemical sunscreen

  - Moisturizers: emollients, humectants, and occlusives

  - Cleansers: non-abrasive, gentle, and pH-balanced

  - Antioxidants: Vitamin C, vitamin E, green tea, glutathione peroxidase, superoxide dismutase and catalase, glutathione (GSH), uric acid, alpha-lipoic acid, ubiquinol

  - Lip balm with sunscreen

A quick note is that, for children younger than 6 months old, it is recommended to avoid sun exposure and not to use any sunscreen. Young children also do not need to use skin cream with too many antioxidants in it because their bodies produce enough antioxidants already. They will benefit from a good moisturizer. It is best to use good nutrition to provide antioxidants and anti-inflammatory ingredients for young children.

Once you see the signs of aging (wrinkles or blemishes) – 2ⁿᵈ line intervention

The first line intervention recommendations are crucial when it comes to looking after your skin and preventing the signs of premature aging. They are really important when it comes to the skincare decisions you must make for your skin today and in the future. When you are young, it is easier to make a big difference in the condition of your skin for the rest of your life. Make sure that you consider all of those first line intervention recommendations carefully.

The second line of intervention is for those who are starting to see signs of aging or who already suffer from aging skin due to intrinsic and/or extrinsic factors. Lifestyle changes are things you can make right now that will stop or even possibly reverse the signs of aging. Knowing what types of products and ingredients to use to help your skin will allow you to make the right decision when it comes to choosing what's best for your skin.

- **Lifestyle changes** (These differ slightly from the ones in the prevention section of this book; I recommend you adopt both sets of lifestyle changes.):

  - Get quality sleep when you cannot get the number of recommended hours of sleep.

  - Use an effective moisturizer: This is especially important for those who must limit their water intake.

- Eat more proteins, get your vitamin B, and calcium, in addition to antioxidants and anti-inflammatory foods: For those who are menopausal, food that contains phytoestrogens is recommended.

- Exercise to increase muscle mass: whole body and facial exercises.

- **Ingredients and products used to treat aging skin:**

  - Sunscreen, moisturizer, cleanser, lip balm: same as in the prevention section of this book

  - Antioxidants: vitamin C, vitamin E, green tea, vitamin A

  - Peptides

  - Vitamin B3

  - Hyaluronic acid

  - Exfoliants: hydroxy acids (AHA, BHA, PHA, BA) and salicylic acids

  - Skin-lightening ingredients: vitamin A, vitamin B3, hydroquinone, salicylic acid, hydroxy acids, alpha-lipoic acid, arbutin, kojic acid

- **Other ways to treat your skin:**

  - Hormone replacement therapy (HRT): Use with caution and discuss with your primary care physician; best to eat food with phytoestrogens

- Microdermabrasion

When the 1st and 2nd lines of intervention fail – the last line of intervention

The last-line option for treating aging skin involves the more invasive treatments that we looked at earlier in the book. They include the things that can have profound side effects, so they need to be undertaken with caution. They are more often than not carried out by a dermatologist or a plastic surgeon and should only be undertaken with counseling and a full understanding of the procedure being carried out. They can have positive effects on the appearance of the skin, but they carry risks with them as well. These include:

- Dermal fillers

- Laser Skin Resurfacing

- Botox injections

- Light/laser therapies

- Dermabrasion

- Non-ablative laser rejuvenation

- Cosmetic surgeries (face lift, neck lift, eye brow lift, and the like)

Prevention of Aging Skin

Lifestyle changes:

- Avoid extreme temperature
- Avoid UV radiation
- Avoid pollution
- Quit smoking and avoid cigarette smoke
- Maintain good nutrition: antioxidants and anti-inflammatory foods
- Get adequate sleep
- Increase water intake – maintain hydration
- Decrease alcohol intake
- Decrease stress

Ingredients and products used to prevent aging skin:

- Sunscreen
- Moisturizers
- Cleansers
- Antioxidants: vitamin C, vitamin E, green tea, glutathione peroxidase, superoxide dismutase and catalase, glutathione (GSH), uric acid, alpha-lipoic acid, ubiquinol
- Lip balm with sunscreen

Treatment of Aging Skin

Lifestyle changes:

- Same as in prevention section
- Get quality sleep; be careful with liquid intake, take in more proteins, vitamin B, and calcium in addition to antioxidants and anti-inflammatory foods
- Exercise and increase muscle mass

Ingredients and products used to treat aging skin:

- Same as prevention: sunscreen, moisturizer, cleanser, lip balm
- Antioxidants: vitamin C, vitamin E, green tea, vitamin A
- Peptides
- Vitamin B3
- Hyaluronic acid
- Exfoliants: hydroxy acids (AHA, BHA, PHA, BA) and salicylic acids
- Skin-lightening ingredients

Other ways to treat

- HRT (with caution) or phytoestrogen-rich food, if menopausal
- Microdermabrasion

Invasive Procedures

- Dermal fillers
- Laser Skin Resurfacing
- Botox injections
- Light/Laser therapies
- Dermabrasion
- Non-ablative laser rejuvenation
- Cosmetic surgeries (face lift, neck lift, eye brow lift, etc.)

MY FINAL ADVICE

Let me leave you with some parting recommendations:

- Don't use products that don't show all the ingredients or try samples that you haven't researched the ingredients of.

- Buy your skincare products from a reputable company with good manufacturing practices.

- Buy for the ingredients, not because of the packaging, the brand, social media or other advertising, or celebrity endorsement.

- Look for products that show you exact percentages of the ingredients you need, if possible.

- Choose the right moisturizer, based on your skin type.

- Just because it's labeled "organic" doesn't mean it's safe.

- Recognize that everything is a chemical. Even water is a chemical that's made up of oxygen and hydrogen. There are "naturally occurring" chemicals and "synthetic" chemicals. You want to use "naturally occurring" chemicals and stay away from synthetics. When a product's label says it's "chemical free", that's false advertising. Everything is made up of chemicals.

- Test products, even if they're labeled "hypoallergenic". To test, dab a small amount of the product on your inner forearm twice a day for four or five days. If you do not have a reaction, it is likely safe for you to apply the product to your face.

- Stop using products that sting or burn unless they were prescribed by a dermatologist. In that case, consult with the dermatologist first before you stop using the product because, for some prescriptions stinging or irritation are expected or considered typical side effects.

- Limit the number of products you use. Using too many products on your skin, especially more than one anti-aging product, can cause irritation. This often makes the signs of aging more noticeable.

- Use a product that can address multiple concerns (for example, sunscreen + moisturizer all in one or antioxidant + sunscreen + moisturizer).

- Create a daily skincare routine: The key to success with most skincare products is repetition because most anti-aging cream takes time to work.

- Apply cream right after the skin is clean and moist. This is when the skin can absorb all the good ingredients you are providing.

- Give the product time to work. When it comes to anti-aging, most products take at least six weeks to work, and some can take up to three months.

- Use products as directed. Applying more than directed can cause clogged pores, a blotchy complexion, irritation or other unwanted effects. Applying too little will not get you the desired effect you're looking for.

- The following are prohibited or restricted cosmetic ingredients by the FDA. Don't buy products that contain these ingredients:

Prohibited Cosmetic Ingredients	CFR Citation
Bithional	21 CFR 700.11
Vinyl chloride	21 CFR 700.14
Certain halogenated salicylanilides	21 CFR 700.15
Zirconium in aerosol products	21 CFR 700.16
Chloroform	21 CFR 700.18
Methylene chloride	21 CFR 700.19
Chlorofluorocarbon propellants	21 CFR 700.23
Prohibited cattle material	21 CFR 700.27
Restricted Cosmetic Ingredients	**CFR Citation**
Mercury compounds	21 CFR 700.13
Hexachlorophene	21 CFR 250.250

And, finally, here are some places on the web where you can get more reliable and unbiased information:

- For reliable, unbiased general health consumer information: Medline Plus: https://medlineplus.gov/

- For more information about cosmetics and their regulation: The FDA's Cosmetics section at: http://www.fda.gov/Cosmetics/default.htm

- For reliable information about natural supplements: Natural Medicines Comprehensive Database at: http://naturaldatabase.therapeuticresearch.com/hom e.aspx?cs=&s=ND (subscription is required)

- For information about different dermatologic procedures: American Society for Dermatologic Surgery at: http://www.asds.net/Home.aspx

- For unbiased clinical and research articles: Pubmed: http://www.ncbi.nlm.nih.gov/pubmed

- For information on certain cosmetic ingredients and why and how to use them, you can check out these websites:

  - http://www.makingcosmetics.com/

  - http://www.paulaschoice.com/cosmetic-ingredient-dictionary/

  - cosmeticsinfo.org

I came across a young lady at a social event who was only 23 years old. She expressed to me that she was concerned with the wrinkles that had started to form on her forehead, and she was considering Botox injections. Now that you have read my book, what do you think my response to her was?

I first asked her if she tried using anything for her wrinkles and whether she had any habits that could contribute to premature aging. At 23, she is too young to consider Botox injections when there are many things she can try first.

I bet that's what you guessed I said, right?

Unfortunately, social media and the prevalence of Botox injections and other such fads currently "trending" are what's being marketed. I hope that, after reading this book, you will be able to help yourself, as well as others, make skincare choices that will help you and they age gracefully without having to resort to drastic measures.

If you have any questions about the content of this book or regarding your skincare regimen, feel free to contact our pharmacy at www.pleasantcarepharmacy.com. Our email address is info@pleasantcarepharmacy.com, and our phone number is 510-200-9984.

ABOUT THE AUTHOR

Let me introduce myself to you by starting with a quote that has motivated me throughout my life and my professional career.

"Better to stop short than to fill to the brim.

Over-sharpen the blade, and the edge will soon blunt.

Amass a store of gold and jade, and no one can protect it.

Claim wealth and titles, and disaster will follow.

Retire when the work is done.

This is the way of heaven."

by Lao Tsu

This quote was the motivation for me to write this book and has inspired me to help people learn to make the right decisions for their skincare needs. It is as simple as this: I feel that this book needs to be written, that I am the right one to do it, and that the time to do it is now.

I do not seek fame or want to increase my financial wealth by writing this book. In fact, all the profits from this book will be donated to the HK Fund, which sponsors low-income people who need eczema or acne cream from Pleasant Care Pharmacy.

Let me tell you a little bit about how the HK Fund came to be. First of all, you should know that the fund's name is made up of the two initial letters in my sons' names – Hieu and Khang.

Hieu began experiencing severe eczema when he was only three months old. Before having my compounding pharmacy, I took him to see different doctors (allergists, dermatologists, naturopathics, and the like), and most of them recommended steroid creams. Some methods I was given to try even made his eczema worse.

As a pharmacist, I knew that using steroid cream long term has many bad side effects. I saw this played out with my son's eczema. So, I created a cream to help control his condition.

Soon, I was able to offer my eczema cream to help others. But, as is always the case with remedies, there was a catch. Because my cream is considered a cosmetic, it is not covered by insurance.

And that is how the HK Fund was born. Creating the fund and writing the book is my way of "paying it forward" to the human community. The monies raised by the HK Fund will help those who need the kind of long-term relief that my eczema cream offers but who cannot afford it.

Now let me tell you about myself and how I came to specialize in the treatment of skin diseases and customized skincare. From a medical credentials standpoint, I received my Bachelor's in Biochemistry, Master of Science in Pharmacology and Toxicology, and a Doctorate degree in Pharmacy. I am currently the co-president of Peninsula Pharmacists Association and the show host of "Pharmacy in Our Lives," a Vietnamese talk show that discusses various health topics from the perspective of a pharmacist.

From a personal standpoint, I have already told you about my son's struggles with eczema and my desire, as his mother, to relieve his pain. So, you see, it is through my own quest to resolve my son's eczema condition that I find myself involved in the treatment of skin disease.

The woman next to me in the picture on the cover of this book is my seventy-seven-year-old grandmother. I hope to look like her when I'm her age. Because we are Asians, we were born with good genes that support antiaging. However, we still need effective skincare solutions to maintain our skin's youthful look. And now that I am involved with customized skincare, my family, including my grandma, are my loyal customers.

In developing my own anti-aging cream, I have learned a lot about the "secrets" to anti-aging, and I am excited to share these with you.

Made in the USA
San Bernardino, CA
18 October 2016